WINNING
SKIN

WINNING
SKIN

The Complete Guide
To Skin Care and Medical Aesthetics

For Skin Care Professionals and Patients

Dean Michael Tomasello, M.D.

Anti-Aging | Medical Aesthetics | Dermatology
The Medical College of Wisconsin

This book is dedicated to those in search of a clear plan to looking and feeling younger and to skin care professionals who strive every day to make their clients achieve the beautiful and youthful appearance they desire.

Contents

Chapter Eight ~ 157
Anti-Aging Laser (and other) Treatments

Chapter Nine ~ 195
Skin Types, Skin Diseases & Aging Eyes

Chapter Ten ~ 233
Beauty and the Future

A note to the reader

In Winning Skin you will learn literally everything you need to know about how skin care and medical aesthetics can effectively make your appearance more youthful, vibrant and beautiful. This book is written for both skin care professionals *and* patients. The concepts discussed herein are easier to incorporate into your life and anti-aging plan than you may have imagined.

Looking and feeling more youthful and beautiful is well within your reach. At its core, Winning Skin is about empowering you. This book comes following my 22 year experience in the areas of anti-aging, skin care, medical aesthetics and wellness. I have educated, mentored and trained countless doctors, nurses, aestheticians and other health professionals. A strength I have is the ability to explain complicated issues in a manner which is understandable to all.

Knowledge is power. It brings confidence and reduces fear and anxiety. The world of skin care, medical aesthetics and anti-aging continues to grow and may seem overwhelming to fully grasp. Winning Skin allows you to master these concepts very well indeed. This book will lead you a full understanding and knowledge of how to easily, effectively, safely and consistently reverse the aging process. Though this you will experience amazing improvements to your skin, your body and your life.

Please note, however, that the contents of Winning Skin should not be considered *medical advice* per se. If you use any ingredients or receive any treatments mentioned in this book and feel as though you are experiencing an allergy or serious side effect, please stop immediately and call 911 or visit the nearest emergency room.

Be good to yourself and your skin.

Dean M. Tomasello, M.D.

Introduction

To have 'Winning Skin' means when you look in the mirror you smile. If you aren't smiling now, by the end of this book you will know exactly what to do to bring a smile every time. For those of you who are pleased with your reflection in the mirror, this book will make certain you stay that way.

Our skin works diligently and tirelessly for us. It connects us to the external environment through nerve endings while regulating temperature and providing a barrier to viruses, bacteria, fungi, allergens and other external threats. It is our body's largest organ and is necessary to our survival; however, it is quite frequently taken for granted.

So how does that smooth and perfect skin we have as a baby become the blemished and wrinkled skin of middle age? These changes don't happen overnight. Through the years these transformations are inevitable if we do not attempt to arrest them.

The skin's regenerative processes slow down as we age. The top layer (epidermis) of the skin does not refresh itself as quickly and has fewer oil glands in middle age as it did in our teens. This makes our skin appear dull and tired. Wrinkles begin to appear and deepen through the years. The lower layers (dermis and subcutaneous layer) become thinner and lose firmness. These changes are all part of the normal aging process. Exposure to UV rays and free radicals hasten this aging process. If we simply stand by and watch, these changes will continue to occur and progress. Without intervention, we will consistently look older every year.

Winning Skin illustrates clearly that these aging factors are by no means inevitable. They can be <u>stopped and reversed</u>. Changes can be made to shift the aging process to an anti-aging course. Winning Skin is your anti-aging path to beauty. I am excited to share it with you.

We will begin by discussing how to recognize the beauty you have. Understanding and developing your self-image is of utmost importance. Though this, you will be on the right track as you move forward in this anti-aging journey. Winning Skin will walk you through the key ingredients and procedures needed to improve each layer of your skin.

Skin care ingredients and aesthetic procedures are effective means to attaining a young and vibrant appearance however, equally meaningful is our diet. Blood flow reaches the layers of the skin through small capillaries. With the right diet, we can deliver high-power antioxidants and other key ingredients through the bloodstream into our skin. Here we are literally helping our skin from the inside-out.

Medical aesthetic procedures such as Botox, dermal fillers and cosmetic laser treatments will be discussed in depth. These are the icing on the cake. Understanding which of these procedures is best for each area of concern will help you be certain that the procedure you choose will bring the most cost-effective, beautiful and natural result.

You will notice as you read through this book that there will be a recurrence of certain anti-aging concepts and a rhythm to them. This is intended to help you fully absorb and retain vitally important anti-aging information and keep it at the forefront of your mind. Through reading this book you will gain a full understanding of the simple, straightforward process to looking and feeling younger. This is what anti-aging is all about.

Regardless of your age or experience with anti-aging, skin care or medical aesthetics, this book is certain to give you a deeper understanding and empower you. Through this, you will be ready to make simple, consistent changes that will make you look and feel more young and beautiful than ever before.

Dean M. Tomasello, MD

Chapter One

Begin To Think Beautiful Now

Many years ago, Michelangelo was asked to elaborate regarding a depiction of a woman he had painted in the Sistine Chapel. He described her as, "worthy of admiration simply because she exists; perfection and imperfection together." There is great power in his statement. It should make you stop and think. This quote came from a man who has been admired for his depiction of beautiful women for over 500 years. Did the woman Michelangelo painted feel beautiful? He certainly appeared to think so.

Self-criticism is like a disease. Countless women stare into the mirror with a relenting need to analyze every blemish, spot, discoloration, line, wrinkle, scar or other *perceived* imperfection. It brings forth feelings of discomfort, helplessness and even utter disgust. Many women who are truly beautiful fail miserably in their ability to recognize it.

Why did I enter the profession of skin care and medical aesthetics? First and foremost, my goal was to help people look and feel more beautiful and youthful. Secondly, medical aesthetics afforded me a profession through which I could express my love of art and all things beautiful. However, I soon realized there was a daunting challenge ahead. Even with the multitude of skin care ingredients and medical aesthetic procedures available, I had a limitation. Despite strides I made to enhance one's personal beauty ... *perceived* imperfections commonly remained. This was a most unwelcome obstacle indeed. Everyone does not have a need to focus on their imperfections. Those who look in the mirror and love what they see are quite fortunate. The reality is that many more are not quite so satisfied.

We have all heard 'beauty is in the eye of the beholder.' However, what if **you** are the beholder and your reflection in the mirror does not look beautiful to you?

Where does this struggle originate? It is my belief that it can be summarized quite simply:

You are not to blame for being critical of your appearance ... you have been *programmed* to be this way.

Understandably, those delving into the realms of skin care, medical aesthetics and anti-aging for the first time may be overwhelmed. There is ongoing research, new products and improved treatments every year. Even the savvy skin care expert may be challenged to keep up-to-date. While this book will explore every nuance to *looking* younger, the idea of *feeling* younger needs to be addressed at the outset. You see, there are countless ways to make you look younger. *Feeling* younger is another story. Sophia Lauren said it best when she noted:

"Nothing makes a woman more beautiful than the belief she is beautiful."

I have dedicated my professional life to helping people (primarily women) look more beautiful and *presumably* feel more beautiful. However, anyone involved in the medical aesthetics profession, from clinic manager to aesthetician to doctor *knows* that improving outer beauty does not equate to *an inner feeling* of beauty.

Why does one woman come into the office, receive a simple treatment, check the mirror and say *"fabulous!"* and walk out smiling while others struggle? Some are never satisfied with their appearance no matter how extensively or frequently they receive treatments.

When you see a beautiful woman, do not immediately assume she feels as lovely as you perceive her to be. This begs the next question. Which is more important? How beautiful *you* think she is or how beautiful *she* thinks she is? I submit to you that her self-perception outweighs any other. In fact, my experience is that someone who is considered gorgeous by most, quite commonly is unable to see the beauty the rest find quite obvious.

Our self-image develops through a complicated interplay between cultural ideas, life experiences, the media and accumulated comments by others. The end result is not necessarily a distortion of reality, it is *our* reality. Studies have shown that generally a person first focuses on a central area of the face (eyes, nose and mouth) of someone they meet or when viewing a picture of an unknown individual. However, every person does not focus on the exact same area. Where a person's eyes are drawn to when looking at another has a great deal to do with their past experiences. Put another way, it has to do with how they have been programmed.

If a young girl was teased about having a big nose, regardless of how beautiful she is as an adult, chances are she is going to check her nose when she looks in the mirror. When she meets someone new, her eyes will focus on that person's nose. She will compare and she will suspect others are staring at her nose as well. She has a negative self-image fixated on her nose.

As another example, women who suffered through years of acne as a teen will understandably become unsettled with a new pimple. One woman is focused on a pimple and another focused on her nose. Some feel this can simply be just chalked up as 'human nature.' My feeling is that it goes much deeper. People are not *born* with self-image issues. They are learned. Sure, my goal is to help you to look and feel younger. The point is, looking younger *and feeling younger* doesn't always go hand in hand. Changing one's self perception is what is needed. The good news is that this change is quite possible, in fact ***probable*** once you become aware of it.

When you meet someone, or look at a picture of them you are seeing a single moment in time. In their mind lies a culmination of every positive or negative comment received throughout their lifetime, their learned ideas of what is beautiful, and an innate need to compare their beauty with that of others. Vanderbilt University psychologist, David Schlundt notes, "All of your experiences, all the teasing you went through as a child, all the self-consciousness you had as a teenager, and all the worrying about whether you would be accepted as good enough or attractive enough are called forth in how people think of themselves."

Dr. Vivian Diller, a psychologist and past Wilhelmina model who treats X-dancers and models agrees, "Your upbringing and the criticisms you heard as a child set a strong foundation for your self-perception in adulthood." Conversely, those who believe themselves to be beautiful may not be considered so at all by society's standards. Chances are, in the formative years these people received a steady diet of positive feedback from friends and loved ones. Your self-image is, in part, a product of your environment.

The point to remember is that everyone has beauty. But beware; the beauty you have is under attack. You are continually being re-programmed to think you need to be more beautiful than you are. This is not your fault either. But, there is something you can do about it. In order for you to feel beautiful about yourself, it is of paramount importance that you become aware of what *around you* is literally attacking your sense of inner beauty. The multi-billion dollar cosmetic, skin care and hair industries are well aware that many people do not feel beautiful *enough*. This comes at you in many forms; the media (including social media), the corporate world and the society in which you live.

Imagine opening up a copy of Cosmopolitan or Vogue magazine. There is an image of a woman poised to sell you a product or service. Let's say it is an anti-aging moisturizer. She is blemish, wrinkle and age spot free with a radiant and glowing face. She will have a flat stomach, thin legs and her weight will be 25% less than the average weight of a US female (For the record in the US = 5 Ft. 4 and 166 lbs.). What is the message? *Buy this product and look like her.* You use the product and while it might help, most women are not going to look like 'her'. If you do not, the next plan recommended is to consider a more expensive option (or simply to buy more). You should get the picture here. Namely, the corporate world does not want you to feel completely satisfied with your looks. You are exposed to this repeatedly over and over until you literally become programmed into believing that you need to look more beautiful than you are.

Nobody goes to see a Star Wars movie and leaves worrying that Darth Vader is going to attack them in the parking lot. It's fantasy. It's not real. The advertisements you see of perfect faces and bodies are, in many ways, fantasy as well. I know I will never be as handsome as Elvis or Cary Grant, but I can make strides to move in that direction. Moving in the right direction is good. Expecting to fully get there along with the body of Michelangelo's David, is setting me up for disappointment. I know that. Try your best to know it too. Advertisements are someone trying to sell you something. Realize it and absorb it. You don't see these people on your typical day walking through the grocery store, mall or coffee shop. If you did, you and everyone around you may do a double take.

In the 21st century social media comes at us as well. We are all exposed to a barrage of social media images that many of us were not when we were teens. Facebook, Instagram and Twitter are part of our psyche and are chuck-full of more images for us to look at and compare ourselves to. These platforms are perfect venues for women to show others how beautiful they are. Many are on the edge of their seat to see how many 'likes' they receive. This can help some feel beautiful, and others feel less so. National Institutes of Health researcher, Heather Patrick states, "We compare how we think we look to how other people look, and make a decision about whether we're much better or much worse."

When it comes to getting a job, beauty matters bigtime. Whether the hiring manager admits to it or not is immaterial. In a study performed in St. Louis, researchers looked at perceived beauty vs. income. People perceived as 'beautiful' made 14% more than those felt to be unattractive. However, this study did not take into account the specifics of 'beauty.' Did you ever see someone who was truly beautiful but who was also shy and insecure with poor posture? That person did not recognize her own beauty. It wasn't shining through. Next, think of a person who is perhaps less attractive yet walks with confidence, smiles a lot with a bubbly and optimistic attitude. Which do you think an employer would *perceive* as more beautiful?

I began my career as a family physician where we are taught to treat the entire person. Many come to a doctor's office or medical spa in an attempt to enhance their beauty and/or attain a more youthful appearance. There is nothing wrong with this at all. Having the right skin care regimen or medical aesthetic procedure can make a world of difference. Unlike many skin care professionals, I do not stop there. Let's take it a step further. After you have had a procedure or treatment to make your appearance more aesthetically pleasing, let's look at how we can allow that outer beauty to seep inside.

When I first studied issues related to negative self-image, I found many of the plans or 'techniques' to be downright silly. However, this two-step approach has been helpful to countless individuals with this issue. I use it myself.

1. Identify Negative Inner Dialogue:

On a typical day people interact with many others and hear varied opinions. We are bombarded with advertisements on billboards, magazines, newspapers, television and the internet. Many of these have to do with beauty.

Ask yourself:

1.   What did I see or hear today that made me question my beauty?
2.   What thoughts did I have?
3.   What feelings arose? Did it make me happy? Angry? Sad? Disappointed? Anxious?
4.   How often do I notice this in a typical day?

2. Replace It:

If that inner dialogue is telling you things such as, "I am not pretty enough" or "I will never be as beautiful as _____," replace it with something positive.

This may seem trite or silly (I thought it was the first time I tried it), but study after study as shown that what we tell ourselves has an immense impact on many aspects of our life. It improves posture, sleep and productivity while reducing fear, depression and anxiety.

Ask yourself: "What is good about you? Are you a good friend? Devoted mother? Valued employee?" And … "What do you like about your appearance?" Beauty may be in the eye of the beholder but if the beholder is you and you don't like what you see in the mirror, we need to change something. The best results are changes to the outside *and* inside.

Never underestimate how powerful this inner dialogue can be. It is estimated that we have internal dialogue or 'self-talk' with ourselves over a thousand times a day. Can you imagine the impact nothing but positive self-talk could have on your outlook on life if you were able to do it? There are many ways that negative self-talk literally can freeze us.

1. It can keep us in an unhealthy relationship. A person may feel as though they are not 'good enough' to be with someone who loves, adores and respects them. Baloney!
2. It tells us that promotion or raise we deserve for working tirelessly for years at a company should not be asked for.
3. Trying something new? Those with a great deal of negative self-talk are not going to rock the boat there.
4. How about buying a beautiful or sexy new outfit? Shut the negative self-talk up and buy it already!

Continued negative self-talk is your enemy and is quite frankly unhealthy. It accomplishes nothing. It prevents you from being the best you can be. My suggestion is that when this nasty inner dialogue tries to take a hold of your psyche, identify it and replace it with something … **anything** positive. It is like throwing water on a tiny fire before it gains momentum and literally burns up your self-image. You are beautiful … don't forget it.

Now let's learn how to make you look and feel more beautiful and younger than ever.

Chapter Two

The Skin and Its Needs

The first point to consider when taking care of your skin is to fully understand what it needs. Your anti-aging plan need not be complicated. A complex skin care plan can be difficult to follow and hugely frustrating. In fact, one of the primary reasons people do not reach their full 'beauty potential' is because they feel it will either be too difficult or too expensive. Neither is true.

Keep it Simple

When it comes to anti-aging, it is best to think of the skin simply and layer by layer. Most every skin care, anti-aging or aesthetic procedure is aimed at helping one or more specific skin factors. I put these into three basic categories. The first step in anti-aging is to understand what each layer is composed of and what we need to do to help that area 'act' younger.

Category 1 – The Epidermis

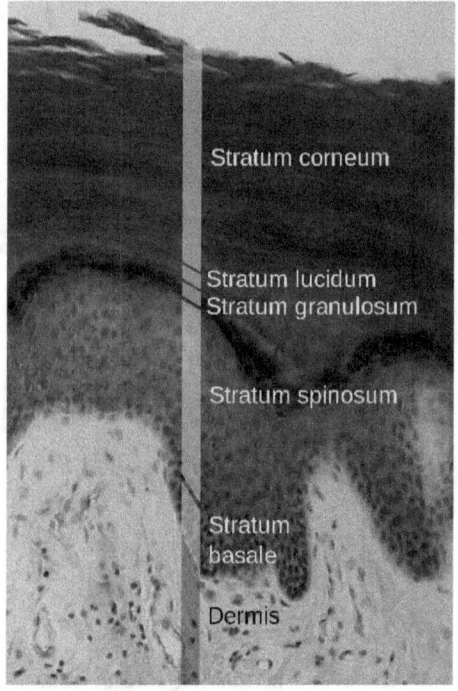

The epidermis is the outermost skin layer composed of five distinct areas. New cells come from the bottom (stratum basale) and move upward until they reach the top (stratum corneum) layer. This top layer is composed of dead cells that serve many protective and moisture-retaining functions. In regard to the epidermis, anti-aging products and treatments should:

1. Clear excess dead skin cells from the skin surface (stratum corneum).
2. Stimulate new cell growth from the stratum basale.
3. Neutralize free radicals.

Category 2 – The Dermis

The dermis is below the epidermis. Here collagen and elastin are of utmost importance. In this layer, cells called *fibroblasts* make collagen and elastin. 70% of the dermis is made up of collagen. Think of collagen and elastin as 'architecture' supporting the epidermis. In order to have beautiful and youthful skin you need a soft and smooth epidermis supported well by a healthy dermis. Collagen and elastin in the dermis keep the skin tight, elastic and firm. Effective products and treatments that help the dermis will:

1. Stimulate fibroblasts to make more collagen and elastin.
2. Clear free radicals that can break down collagen and elastin.
3. Improve the function or prevent breakdown of collagen and elastin through the use of neurotoxins and dermal fillers. More collagen and elastin equates to tighter and firmer skin.
4. Improve blood flow to the dermis. The blood flow in the dermis supplies oxygen and nutrients to both the dermis and epidermis.

Category 3 – Moisture and UV Protection

This is an important maintenance category. The skin needs to be nurtured and protected. Hydrated skin is youthful and happy skin. Avoid stripping protective oils and keep the skin well hydrated. Block UV rays from your skin as much as possible. These rays cause the formation of hefty amounts free radicals in both the epidermis and dermis resulting in premature skin aging.

How Neurotoxins (like Botox) and Dermal Fillers Fit into Category 2

Neurotoxins (i.e. Botox, Dysport and Xeomin) inhibit facial muscle movement. Every time you yawn, smile, laugh, squint or frown, the small muscles around the eyes, brow and forehead repeatedly contract and squeeze the skin (and collagen) between them. With continued movement, fine lines and wrinkles form and deepen. This is most noticeable around the eyes (crow's feet), brow (between the eyebrows) and the forehead. The anti-aging effects of neurotoxins occur due to a temporary block of these facial muscles.

Botox does more than just stop muscle movement though; it goes a step further. A study in the *JAMA Facial Plastic Surgery* (May 2015) showed that Botox increased the stretch and elastic recoil in the skin of women studied. This mimicked younger skin. Therefore, by relaxing the muscles, you now literally have less wear and tear on the collagen and elastin. Yes, Botox relaxes facial muscles, however it also gives collagen and elastin a chance to stretch out and strengthen. Through this, we are improving the strength and elasticity of the dermis. Our supporting architecture is improved. Therefore, Botox brings powerful anti-aging power beyond what was originally thought.

Dermal Fillers (i.e. Restylane, Juvederm, and Radiesse) do more than just 'fill in' wrinkles. If the injector is skilled, the dermal filler will both fill in the area of deficit as well as stimulate the growth of collagen and elastin. A large 'bolus' injection of a filler into a wrinkle is not optimal. Spreading the filler out during the injection (commonly referred to as 'fanning') is best.

1. Spreading the filler out presents the dermis with a larger product 'surface area.' For hyaluronic acid fillers like Restylane, this means a greater moisture-retaining potential. For a product like Radiesse, it means a larger collagen stimulating area.

2. The process of spreading the filler out also serves to cause a greater stimulation of collagen-producing fibroblasts in the dermis. It is true that the injection itself can elicit anti-aging effects.

There are countless products and treatments which can help your skin look younger. It is important to remember to keep it simple. With each product used or procedure performed, be aware of which category is going to benefit most. Having this awareness will be of great benefit to you in accomplishing your anti-aging goals.

How Our Skin Ages

As you transition from your early twenties into your fifties, your face lets you know. There are many factors that contribute to the way our face ages. These can be easily identified. The good news is that the list of anti-aging skin care ingredients and procedures continues to grow and become more accessible to everyone. You will learn about these in the chapters that follow. Twenty years ago, most people felt visiting the cosmetic surgeon was the only option. Indeed it was. Granted, cosmetic surgeons can make amazing surgical changes to your face to shed 5-10 years (or more) off. Today many of these same surgeons also employ non-surgical options which are cost effective ways to bring beautiful and youthful results. For this and many other reasons, medical aesthetics has a rock-solid presence in the anti-aging realm.

Age and Your Face

Age 20-29

Largely, this is the 'life is good' decade. In the epidermis your skin is cranking out new, fresh and vibrant cells at a beautiful clip. The rate of cell turnover of new cells being formed at the basal layer of the epidermis to the top (stratum corneum) layer is 24-28 days. This means the appearance of fine lines or wrinkles is rare. With a little regular exfoliation and some moisturizing the skin surface remains smooth and gorgeous. In the dermis, there is plenty of collagen and elastin to support the epidermis. Soaking up UV rays elicits a quick response from vibrant melanocytes revealing a polished and velvety tan. The moisture level in the skin is optimal along with a plump and full subcutaneous fat layer (below the dermis). These factors all contribute to a smooth and youthful appearance to the skin of those in their 20s.

Age 30-39

Life is still pretty good but the aging signs begin to arrive. That excessive sunbathing from earlier years rears its ugly head. About 25% of your lifetime sun exposure occurs by age 18. This exposure is cumulative and now you have had 30+ years of it. The melanin begins to form clumps and is now less evenly distributed. Ultimately age spots and other areas of increased skin pigment in the epidermis begin to show up. Women who have had a lot of UV exposure, had become pregnant or used birth control are at an increased risk to develop melasma. UV exposure increases the presence of collagenase, an enzyme that breaks down collagen. You are ten years older now with another decade of the cumulative effects of free radical exposure. These come from UV rays, your diet, dust, smoking, allergens, heat, cold and pollution. The skin has less moisture and while new vibrant epidermal cells are continually coming to the surface as they did in your 20s, this rate has slowed.

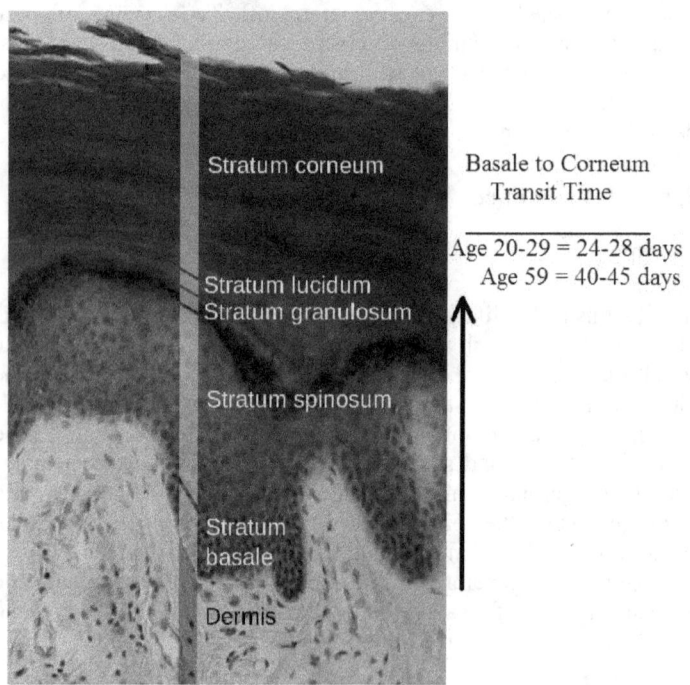

Stratum corneum

Stratum lucidum
Stratum granulosum

Stratum spinosum

Stratum basale

Dermis

Basale to Corneum Transit Time

Age 20-29 = 24-28 days
Age 59 = 40-45 days

All these factors mean fine lines and wrinkles begin to appear as do inconsistencies in skin tone. Broken blood vessels pop up here and there. It is during this decade that most women come in to see the aesthetician or medical aesthetic doctor to begin an anti-aging plan. In fact, in a survey of 129 women at Dean Michael Aesthetics in 2010, the average age at the first such appointment was 34.

Age 40-50

What is happening here? Gravity is no friend of beauty at any age, but in your 40s it seems like some new G-force pointing south is taking over. If you happen to be going out for a few cocktails and forget your ID, don't worry, nobody is asking for it.

Now the rubber has clearly hit the road. Everything that you disliked about your appearance in your 30s has now done nothing but worsen. Women in their late forties or early fifties get to deal with menopause as well. So what is happening to your skin now? The epidermis is becoming thinner and drier. The blood flow from the dermis that supplies oxygen and nutrients to the skin is less brisk. The rate of turnover of new and vibrant cells from the basal layer to the top epidermal layer continues to slow. The skin has less collagen, elastin and subdermal fat. All these factors mean that the architecture supporting the epidermis has weakened. The skin is more prone to the development of fine lines, wrinkles and the dreaded 'loose skin.'

Age 50+

The reduction of estrogen seen after menopause hits your skin hard. The epidermis becomes even thinner and drier. Blood flow to the dermis becomes sluggish. This results in a reduction in oxygen and nutrient delivery. The repair of collagen and elastin slows down = less firmness to the dermal layer. After age 50 there is a further decrease in subcutaneous fat. There is less protective melanin making your skin more prone to sun damage. This is most noticeable in the face, neck and hands.

I suspect reading though this section may paint a very bleak picture. This progression is typical in the skin of the face *without intervention*. However, as we delve into the world of skin care and anti-aging you will soon understand quite clearly that each of these changes described can be arrested and in most cases reversed. As you learn more about skin care and anti-aging you will quickly realize that this normal age progression is by no means inevitable. Remember to keep a simple and consistent approach with any and all treatments.

Anti-Aging Essentials

If you look at a newborn's perfect skin, you get a clear picture as to what we are up against. The newborn skin is smooth and vibrant without a blemish, wrinkle, sag or spot. It is the type of skin we strive for and what brings us to see skin care professionals. Every year billions of dollars are spent by those attempting to look more beautiful and youthful. Anti-aging and having Winning Skin means loving the skin you are in. Anti-aging essentials are *also* beautiful skin essentials. Although these are not ingredients per se, they are vital to your anti-aging plan.

The internet is a wonderful way to find information and to communicate with others. However, it can work against you when it comes to your search for ways to help your skin. Do not enter 'anti-aging' in the Google search bar. If you do, you will be met with 45 million listings. The vast majority of people look for links on the first page of search results. This means they are getting advertisements and not the best information. The same holds true if you perform a search for the term 'acne.' Here you get 81 million results.

There are many definitions for anti-aging. My definition is:

"Consistent intervention aimed at arresting and reversing the aging process resulting in an internal and external anatomy and physiology more youthful than one's stated age."

Medical aesthetics and cosmetic surgery are viable and effective means to attain a more youthful appearance externally. No argument there. However, I always explain to patients that while the external is important, if you aren't working on the internal, you are missing the big picture. It's icing with no cake.

In the next chapter we discuss key skin care ingredients necessary to help you attain the supple and youthful skin you desire. However, before we proceed, it is vital that you become aware of the following 8 anti-aging essentials.

1. Dietary Free Radicals

You will hear a great deal about antioxidants and free radicals in this book. Free radicals are atoms or groups of atoms with an odd (unpaired) number of electrons. This happens when oxygen interacts with certain molecules. Once formed these highly unstable molecules start a chain reaction like dominoes. The free radical scavenges through your skin looking for another electron. In the process it attacks and damages the cells around it; cell proteins, membranes, the outside of the cell (cytoskeleton), the inside of the cell, even the cell's DNA. Free radicals form in your skin in response to a multitude of environmental factors including UV rays, heat, cold, smoking, pollution, dust, allergens and dietary factors to name a few.

Fatty meats, red meat or meats with preservatives such as bacon, ham, pepperoni, salami, corned beef and other deli meats have ingredients associated with a greater production of free radicals. The National Institutes of Health has shown that free radicals are hard on our arteries (heart disease, stroke), nerves (Alzheimer's, Parkinson's) and can contribute to diabetes. Further, limiting foods with high sugar content is helpful to your skin. Foods with high sugar content are also described as having a high 'glycemic index.' White bread or rice, sugary cereals, potatoes, French fries, scones, muffins and sugary fruit juices or colas all have a high glycemic index.

Antioxidants neutralize free radicals. If you limit the foods associated with free radical formation while consuming more antioxidant-rich foods you are helping your body fight the aging process. Anti-oxidant rich foods contain vitamins A, C, E and Beta Carotene (fruits and vegetables). Other free radical fighters include green tea and resveratrol (which contain polyphenols) and lycopene (in fruits and vegetables).

In chapter 5 we will discuss the Clear Skin Diet which is made up of powerful antioxidant foods while limiting foods that cause the formation of free radicals. Free radical neutralization cannot be stressed enough.

2. Alcohol in Moderation

This one is pretty straightforward. Most of us have heard that one or two glasses of wine a day may have some cardiac benefits. If you are drinking more than this, you are doing nothing but giving your body more free radicals to neutralize. Further, alcohol blocks a hormone produced by your kidneys called *anti-diuretic hormone* (or ADH). By blocking ADH, your kidneys lose more water than they should. This results in dehydration. Hangovers are largely due to dehydration. Further, if you are dehydrated, your skin most certainly is. Our goal is anti-aging. Dehydrated skin with large amounts of free radicals will age the skin prematurely. If you stick with one or two glasses of wine a day, you will receive cardiac benefits without causing adverse effects to your skin.

3. Exercise

When it comes to exercise, there are several factors worth mentioning. First of all, exercise consumes oxygen which will increase the formation of free radicals. During exercise, the body does a very good job of beefing up its own production of antioxidants to combat the oxidative stress and increased free radical load. Supplementing this with dietary antioxidants or antioxidant supplements is helpful here. Unless one is partaking in frequent *extreme workouts* (heart rate over 85% maximal for over 30 minutes), I don't feel that the anti-oxidant formation during exercise should deter anyone from incorporating exercise into their weekly anti-aging plan.

Here is why:

Exercise increases *telomere length*. Telomeres are the caps at the ends of DNA strands that protect the chromosomes in each cell. They are like the plastic tips at the end of shoelaces. Without these telomeres, DNA strands become damaged, do not function efficiently and may die. Moderate exercise has been shown to improve telomeres. These little 'DNA caps' are currently under extensive investigation for the powerful role they play in anti-aging. One study showed that those exercising three hours a week had telomeres that appeared 9 years younger than those who did not exercise. In addition, regular moderate exercise has been shown to have an important role in reducing inflammation throughout the body.

Discuss with your doctor if you plan to incorporate exercise into your wellness and anti-aging plan. In my experience, getting started is the most difficult part. Exercise burns calories and fat, increases telomere length and reduces inflammation while improving the circulation to your skin and other vital organs. People who exercise regularly have also been shown to have improvements in chronic conditions like anxiety, depression and insomnia.

4. Stress Reduction

Those with the most stress in their lives are most likely to fall into unhealthy eating, drinking and sleeping habits. Further, in regard to telomeres, increased work or life stress is associated with *shorter* telomere lengths. Those with less stress have been shown to have *longer* telomere lengths. Shorter telomeres have been linked to the development of Parkinson's disease, type II diabetes, cardiovascular disease and cancer. So saying, "this job is killing me" may not be that far from the truth. Without a doubt it is affecting your telomeres resulting in older and less healthy cell DNA.

The first step is to identify and admit you are stressed out ... and do something about it. Whether you choose reading, yoga, meditation, massage, theatre, movies, spending time with family or physical activity in the form of sports or going to the gym, you *need a stress release.* Some find a hobby. Just knowing that you will have a part of your day that will be relaxing can reduce your overall daily stress. Talking with a therapist, doctor or psychiatrist may help as well. I certainly am not suggesting anyone quit their job, however, if you are in a position to change to a less stressful job, I would strongly recommend it.

5. Get Enough Sleep

Seven to nine hours of sleep per night is vital to the health of your body and skin. Sleep renews and regenerates the skin through increased collagen production and improved moisture. Growth hormones also peak during sleep. These play a key role in cell repair. Lack of sleep weakens the immune system and makes you more prone to viruses. Poor sleep will also aggravate chronic skin conditions like eczema, psoriasis, rosacea and acne. The CDC estimates that one third (33%) of adults age 18-60 do not receive the recommended minimum of 7 hours of sleep per night.

The first part of your face to suffer from lack of sleep is around your eyes. They may appear puffy, baggy with deeper fine lines. The eyes themselves can appear red as well. Your best bet for getting a good night's sleep is to develop and maintain a healthy sleep routine.

- Try to keep a consistent bedtime/awake time schedule.
- Exercise regularly. Muscle fatigue sends signals to your brain telling your body to rest. People who exercise regularly sleep better.
- Keep your bedroom a bit cooler than the rest of your home (2-3 degrees).
- Avoid greasy or sugary foods, alcohol or caffeine after 6 pm.
- Try to develop a 'pre-sleep' ritual (reading, meditation, soft music).
- Make your bedroom a technology-free zone. Watching TV, using a computer or phone before bed can be stimulating and can delay sleep onset.
- If you are aware that you snore, chances are your sleep is interrupted. Speak with your doctor and consider getting a sleep study.
- Speak to a therapist, counselor or psychiatrist about stresses in your life.
- As an absolute last resort, consider medications *under the care of a physician.*

6. Keep Your Skin Well Hydrated

Four to five 16 ounce glasses of water a day is an excellent goal for most. When you are dehydrated your skin suffers. It is dry, secretions are thicker and glands are more easily blocked. I love hyaluronic acid in skin care. When used as a topical agent in the form of serum or moisturizer, the hyaluronic acid attracts water from its environment. It partially sits on the surface serving as a barrier to keep moisture in. Other excellent choices are coconut oil (if no acne) and argan or tea tree oil (if acne is present). There are literally hundreds of quality moisturizers.

This brings up a final point; Make your AM and PM skin care regimen simple and straightforward. Many companies are very interested in having you buy and use 3-5 products several times a day. Simple is better. The role of essential oils and the benefits to your overall skin hydration is discussed in Chapter 3.

7. Don't Smoke

Although an obvious anti-aging measure, I include it here to remind you that smoking/nicotine reduces blood flow to your skin resulting in less collagen and elastin and more fine lines and wrinkles. Studies have shown that smoking actually results in more premature facial aging than UV ray exposure. Quitting smoking puts years onto your life and improves every layer of your skin. If you are a smoker, the biggest change you can make in the anti-aging realm … is to quit.

8. Use Sun Block

Ultraviolet (UV) rays are a type of light ray coming from the sun invisible to the naked eye. When we discuss protecting our skin we need to be aware of three types of UV rays: UVA, UVB and UVC. We don't need to consider UVC rays to any degree since these very short wavelength rays never penetrate the ozone layer of the earth. UVA and UVB are the rays that reach our skin and are responsible for the aging of our skin, sunburn, sun damage (age spots) and in the worst scenario, skin cancers. When these rays hit the skin they alter the skin cell's DNA resulting in damage to the epidermis (top layer) as well as the lower layers of skin. The most important fact regarding UV rays that you need to remember is that they cause the formation of very large amounts of damaging free radicals.

UVA

UVA has the longest wavelength of any UV rays hitting our skin and accounts for 95% of all UV radiation that reaches the earth. The presence of UVA does not change with intensity throughout the year.

These are the rays that sneak up on you on a cloudy day. They are powerful enough to penetrate clouds, clothing and glass. That sunburn you suffered on an overcast day was from UVA rays. I have treated individuals who are in their automobile a great deal of time (i.e. truck drivers). Extended hours of unprotected UVA exposure has resulted in a 'left side of the face' sun damage pattern in these people. UVA rays are powerful and punishing; affecting both the epidermis and dermis. They load the dermis with collagen-destroying free radicals which ultimately leads to wrinkles. Tanning beds are notorious for causing skin damage. This is because they bombard your skin with high doses of UVA rays. When you leave a tanning bed your skin is loaded with free radicals that were not present an hour earlier.

In response to UVA rays, your skin increases melanin production, making your skin darker in an attempt to prevent further damage to the DNA. Someone with a deep dark tan has skin loaded with free radicals and is fighting a war against them due to UVA rays. These rays are so powerful they have even been shown to suppress the immune system.

UVB

UVB rays are a shorter wavelength than UVA and their intensity varies by time of day, season or location. For example, UVB rays are going to be strongest at noon-2pm on a clear day. UVA and UVB can both cause sunburn, skin darkening and premature aging of the skin. UVB is concentrated more-so on the epidermis and will literally cause the skin to 'burn.' Hence, the term *sunburn* is accurate. While both UVA and UVB can cause skin cancers, most experts agree that skin cancers are more commonly related to UVB exposure. While UVA rays hit both the epidermis and dermis, it is the UVB rays that literally 'fry' the epidermal (top) skin surface.

SPF

Did you ever notice some people burn more easily than others? Your natural SPF dictates how long you can stay out in the sun before your skin starts to burn. Fair skinned people have a shorter natural SPF than those with darker skin. The **SPF** designation on sunblock stands for 'Sun Protection Factor.' A product with an SPF of 20 means you can stay out in the sun 20 times longer before your skin begins to burn. A natural SPF of 15 minutes means you will begin to see skin redness after 15 minutes of unprotected UV exposure. Applying SPF 20 sunblock means now the skin will not begin to burn for 20X15 minutes (or 5 hours). If you are going to have UV exposure for 10 hours, the SPF needs to be increased to at least 40, or the SPF 20 needs to be reapplied. I prefer sunblock to sunscreen. Much like a screen door which lets 'some' light through, sunscreen doesn't fully block UVA/UVB rays. Sunblock, on the other hand scatters all of the UV rays so they are completely unable to penetrate the skin. Sunblock typically contains ingredients such as titanium oxide or zinc oxide.

Now that you have an understanding of what your skin needs, how it ages and anti-aging essentials it is time to dig deeper. Remember:

1. The skin care and medical aesthetic measures used externally will indeed help you to have a more youthful appearance. However, making these external changes will have far reaching and deeper results if steps are taken to improve your inner dialogue. We all are beautiful creatures and it is important to find your inner beauty.

2. There are three essential ways (Category 1, 2, 3) that need to be at the forefront of your mind when you are looking to make your appearance more youthful.

   1. Clearing dead cells from the epidermis while stimulating new vibrant cells
   2. Increasing collagen and elastin in the dermis
   3. Blocking UV rays and keeping your skin hydrated

These essential steps are vital if you are serious about anti-aging. Medical aesthetic and surgical procedures can make you quickly more beautiful on the outside. By following preventative measures and working on the inside as well, those external changes will last longer in a body that feels younger. Consistency is the key. Following a simple and reasonable plan is your best bet. The better you are able to follow this plan, the *younger* you will be. Those who are successful with their anti-aging plan consistently ask themselves,

"Is this choice going to make me look and feel younger, or older?"

Chapter Three

Skin Care Ingredients

When it comes to skin care, it is all about ingredients. Through making the best choices you can quickly reach your anti-aging goals. While it is not possible to use every ingredient, it is important to understand each of them. There is a method to the approach as well. Some ingredients should not be mixed and certain ones should be put on your face before others. We will discuss these situations as well.

Skin care products don't always make a point of telling you the important elements in their products. The label "hyaluronic acid moisturizer" is more helpful and descriptive than something like, "age-defying cream." When you see a list of ingredients on a skin care product, pay particular attention to the first third of those listed. These are the additives in the highest concentrations in the product. Since you are buying something that you will be putting on your face, it is important to understand exactly what is in it. Through this understanding, you will be on your way to making ingredient-based strides toward a more youthful appearance.

Think of your skin like you would your heart or lungs. You can check your pulse to determine your heart rate and most certainly can tell your lungs are functioning with every breath you take. Similarly the skin is a living, breathing, constantly renewing organ every minute of every day. It protects us from the external environment and is vital to our survival.

All living organisms have a basic and primary need ...water. Your skin is the most happy when it has plenty of moisture. The average adult's body is composed of at least 60% water and is covered by 15-20 square feet of skin. Without adequate moisture, skin becomes dry and irritated and is more prone to the development of blocked pores, fine lines and wrinkles. Skin diseases such as dermatitis, acne and eczema worsen when the skin is dry. Hyaluronic acid is one ingredient that helps your skin remain moist.

Hyaluronic Acid

It may seem odd that putting something on your skin called "acid" could actually make you look younger but indeed hyaluronic acid most certainly can. Hyaluronic acid is what is known as a *glycosaminoglycan* (glahy-kohs-*uh*-mee-noh-**glay**-kan). For many years I have recommended the use of this go-to skin care ingredient to keep a patient's face supple and moist. This is not just for those with dry skin. Hyaluronic acid is a moisturizer for all skin types. It is a key ingredient necessary to help reduce the presence of fine lines and wrinkles while keeping the skin soft and smooth.

How does hyaluronic acid do this?
Hyaluronic acid is a *humectant*.

A Humectant such as glycerin or hyaluronic acid *attracts* and retains moisture in your skin.

An Occlusive works by forming a thin film on the surface of the skin to *prevent loss* of moisture. It is the occlusive nature of essential oils that allows them to keep the skin moist. They prevent skin moisture from escaping.

An Emollient helps to make the external skin layers more soft and supple. In doing so, they improve hydration and reduce evaporation.

The hyaluronic acid molecules are fairly large, too much so to be fully absorbed through the epidermis. Therefore, they partially sit on the top of the skin keeping the skin moist and serving to a lesser degree as an occlusive. Hyaluronic acid both attracts moisture to your skin while trapping moisture inside.

More moisture = smoother skin = less wrinkles.

Hyaluronic acid dermal fillers such as Juvederm or Restylane are used widely in the field of medical aesthetics. They are injected into areas of the face where wrinkles or volume loss is present. The premise here is quite similar. By injecting the hyaluronic acid into the area of deficit, not only does the filler itself remove wrinkles, but moisture (water) is attracted to the area as well. This allows the area to stay filled in for extended periods of time. In people that stay well hydrated, the dermal filler lasts longer.

Skin care products effective in fighting wrinkles and the natural aging process commonly contain hyaluronic acid. I consider it an ingredient that needs to be a staple of any skin care regimen. It is strongly anti-aging and an efficient wrinkle-fighter.

Hyaluronic acid is a naturally occurring substance in nature in both humans and animals. It is found in skin as well as joint fluid and connective tissues. It lubricates and is fact, quite 'slippery' when present in the body's joints. It has other uses such as wound healing which makes it ideal for use with burn injuries. It is also an excellent moisturizer to be used following certain laser surgeries.

Antioxidants

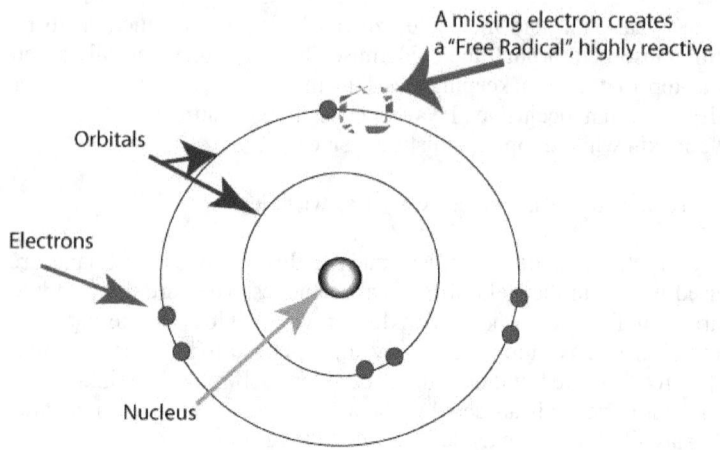

A missing electron creates a "Free Radical", highly reactive

Orbitals

Electrons

Nucleus

Before we discuss antioxidants, let's delve further into free radicals. These are atoms or groups of atoms with an odd (unpaired) number of electrons. A free radical occurs when oxygen interacts with certain molecules. Once formed these highly reactive free radicals start a chain reaction … like dominoes. Free radicals are perhaps more important than any other factor in the realm of anti-aging. If the skin is exposed to more free radicals, it simply ages more quickly.

The free radical scavenges about looking for another electron. In its search it damages anything in its path. This includes cell proteins, membranes, the outside of the cell (cytoskeleton), the inside of the cell and even the cell's DNA is at risk. Free radicals form in your skin in response to a multitude of environmental and dietary factors. Antioxidants neutralize free radicals. In doing so, they also protect and stimulate collagen, aid cell repair and reduce inflammation. Our skin busily makes its own antioxidants and tries desperately to keep up and clear away all the free radicals. Unfortunately it commonly falls short. This is why the addition of antioxidants both in our diet and our skin care regimen is of utmost importance. Through taking these steps, we are helping our skin win the war against free radicals.

Free radicals = bad for skin | Antioxidants = good for skin

In chapter 5 we will discuss how antioxidants in our diet help our bodies and our skin. The free radicals in our skin need to be attacked from the outside (skin care) and the inside (diet/supplements). Antioxidant-containing skin care ingredients are of paramount importance. The following are go-to antioxidants which neutralize free radicals *and* make your skin appear younger in many other ways.

The first antioxidants I list are what can be remembered easily as the "ACE" vitamins; Vitamins A, C and E. When you are looking at ingredients in your skin care regimen or diet, you will never go wrong with the ACE vitamins. These are powerful antioxidants which will keep your skin looking fresh, vibrant and youthful.

Vitamin A (Retinol)

The term 'Vitamin A' is a blanket term for a 'Retinoid' (or Retinol); the biologically active compounds that occur naturally in both animal and plant tissues. Vitamin A has a wide range of uses in our bodies including vision, reproduction, immune function and heart, lung and kidney health.

The term 'Retinoid' is commonly used interchangeably with the term 'retinol' but there is a difference. A Retinoid typically has a higher concentration of the active ingredient *retinoic acid* compared to 'retinol' which is more often associated with lower (over the counter) strength preparations. The semantics here are quite frankly not that important. They are both derivatives of vitamin A. When retinol is put onto the skin it is converted to the 'active' retinoic acid. When I explain the importance of vitamin A to patients, I find it simpler to refer to vitamin A as 'retinol which can come in different strengths.'

The first vitamin A derivative used was *tretinoin*. This is the *carboxylic acid form* of vitamin A and quite powerful. It was FDA approved in 1971 for the treatment for acne under the trade name *Retin-A*. After using Retin-A to treat acne patients for a period of time, dermatologists noticed that these individuals experienced improvements beyond a mere clearing of acne lesions. Their skin was softer and brighter with fewer fine lines. This gave a strong indication that indeed vitamin A did much more than simply clear acne from the skin.

How Retinol Works:

Retinol has been proven in clinical studies to unclog and tighten pores (thereby clearing acne), reverse skin damage due to UV rays, increase blood flow to the skin, boost collagen, even skin tone and speed cell turnover. It is due to this long list of benefits that I have described retinol as 'your skin's best friend' for many years. Using skin care products containing retinol will help your skin become more vibrant and youthful. It is a powerful antioxidant which brings a host of anti-aging strengths.

Vitamin A (retinol) brings anti-aging power through:

- **Combating Hyperkeratinization**

Hyperkeratinization is a disorder of the cells lining the hair follicle. In normal skin, these cells are continually sloughed off, keeping the pores open and the skin clear. In individuals with hyperkeratinization, the cells stagnate and do not leave the follicle due to an excess amount of the protein 'keratin.' This causes a buildup of these cells which ultimately blocks pores. This blockage can be exacerbated further by bacteria that grow well in the moist, closed environment of a blocked pore. The end result is excess dead skin cells, blocked pores and acne or keratosis pilaris (a condition that closely mirrors acne). Retinol battles hyperkeratinization by clearing (exfoliating) the dead skin cells from the pores. This keeps the pores open and reduces the presence of bacteria. It is clear that through this action it is also hugely beneficial to those suffering with acne.

- **Boosting Collagen in Two Ways**

Collagen is what gives our skin its structure, firmness and elasticity. Age and sun exposure break down this collagen resulting in fine lines, wrinkles and sagging skin. When skin is exposed to the UV rays of the sun, there is an increase in *collagenase*. This is an enzyme that literally breaks down collagen. Retinol effectively blocks the collagenase enzyme. With less collagenase, our collagen is far safer.

Retinol, in addition to blocking the collagenase, stimulates an increased *production* of collagen. Hence, in two separate ways, retinol helps our skin's dermal layer have more collagen. The result is smoother skin with fewer fine lines and wrinkles.

- **Increasing Cell Turnover**

Retinol further helps to improve skin texture and fade dark spots or freckles due to its ability to cause cells to turn over more rapidly. The 3-4 week life span of a skin cell is shortened by retinol. New fresh cells are pushed to the skin surface at a faster rate. Quickening the cell turnover rate makes the skin more vibrant and tends to slowly fade unwanted pigment over a period of time.

- **Reducing Inflammation**

Retinol plays a substantial role in blocking the inflammatory response of the skin to different stimuli. This makes the skin less likely to be red or irritated. The anti-inflammatory actions of retinol are particularly helpful to those with acne.

Forms of Prescription Vitamin A:

Prescription Vitamin A	Powerful form of Vitamin A	Primary Uses
Retin- A	Tretinoin	Acne
Renova	Tretinoin	Sun damage/ Anti-aging
Tri-Luma	Tretinoin (and hydroquinone)	Sun damage / Anti-aging
Tazorac	Tazarotene	Acne / Anti-aging
Differin	Adapalene	Acne / Anti-aging

Prescription versions of retinol such as Retin-A, Renova and Tri-Luma contain *tretinoin.* This is the powerful carboxylic acid form of vitamin A. While Retin-A is most commonly used with acne, Renova is regularly prescribed for wrinkles and sun damage. Tri-luma also contains prescription strength hydroquinone and is helpful in the clearing of dark discolorations and melasma. Tazorac contains tazarotene and Differin contains adapalene. These are all powerful, prescription forms of vitamin A.

It is important to remember that while vitamin A (Retin-A) was found initially to clear acne, since that time it has been proven to have multiple effective uses as a topical anti-aging vitamin.

There is great anti-aging power in vitamin A creams and serums available in over-the-counter strengths as well.

Over the Counter Vitamin A:

Over the counter retinol-containing serums or creams are not as potent as their prescription-strength counterparts. However, they do indeed work very well and are less expensive than you may imagine. There are literally hundreds of over the counter preparations available. Studies have shown that even 0.01% retinol has beneficial anti-aging effects on the skin. Typically over-the-counter preparations come as low (< 0.04%) and medium (0.04-.010%) strengths. While these ingredients bring anti-aging power to your skin, they work even better when combined with other ingredients (i.e. vitamin C and vitamin E).

Side Effects and Precautions:

- Retinol can cause dryness, redness and flaking if you start using it too quickly and frequently. For the first two weeks it should be used every third night. If your skin is not irritated you may increase to every other night for the next two weeks and if you are tolerating that well, then continue daily use.
- Wait 10-15 minutes after washing your face before you apply retinol. Let your face literally *calm down* after the washing. Use a very small amount (about a pea size) to cover your face. More than that is not helpful and is more likely to cause irritation. After applying consider following with a moisturizer to prevent dryness. Remember: retinol before moisturizer.
- Use UVA/UVB block with retinol. Since it exfoliates the skin, your skin is a bit more prone to burn following the use of

vitamin A. It does not make your skin any more prone to sun damage than any other type of mild exfoliation. Use a minimum of SPF 30.

- Benzoyl peroxide and alpha hydroxy acids may reduce how effectively retinol performs on your skin. Therefore, you should not layer these products on your face when using retinol.
- Do not use if you are pregnant or nursing.

Vitamin C – (L-Ascorbic Acid)

Vitamin C supplements indeed facilitate optimal health. Vitamin C in pill form helps the skin but not as much so as the use of creams and serums applied directly to the skin. Vitamin C is another good friend to your skin. It beautifully clears free radicals, stimulates collagen (reduces wrinkles), reduces skin discolorations, strengthens the skin's barrier and reduces inflammation. It also helps the skin withstand UV exposure whether sunblock is being applied or not. Vitamin C breaks down on UV and air exposure so should come in a closed container such as a pump.

Vitamin C Beautifies Your Skin:

- It rids our skin of free radicals, those aggressive atoms searching for another electron.

- It stimulates collagen production and strengthens the skin's barrier function.

- It reduces skin discolorations.

- Vitamin C reduces inflammation. Certain chemicals like *arachidonic acid* are present in the skin when it is inflamed. Through chemical pathways, vitamin C blocks the production of arachidonic acid, thereby reducing inflammation in the skin.

- Vitamin C also improves the ability of the skin to withstand UV exposure whether sunblock is being used or not.

The L-ascorbic acid form of vitamin C is water soluble which means it primarily exerts its anti-aging effects on the *inside* of the cell. I mentioned that topical vitamin C is perhaps more beneficial to your skin than dietary vitamin C. In chapter 5 we will discuss in detail how diet can make all these external treatments work better and last longer. Vitamin C is beneficial to health of several important body systems when present in the diet.

- It boosts the immune system through strengthening the body's white blood cells. These cells block viruses and bacteria and comprise a vital part of our body's defense against illness. Further, those who do not get enough vitamin C are more vulnerable to infections, illness and even cancer.

- Vitamin C helps our nervous system produce neurotransmitters. These substances are vital to the ability of nerves to communicate efficiently with one another.

- It assists the production of L-carnitine, an amino acid and building block for proteins. This aids in the transport of fats to the powerhouses of the cell (mitochondria) where they are converted to energy. L-carnitine is vital to many body processes including efficient functioning of the brain, heart and muscles.

Vitamin C-Ester

Taking vitamin C to a whole new level is vitamin C-Ester. This is vitamin C (L-ascorbic acid) joined to the fatty acid *palmitic acid* (derived from palm oil). Vitamin C-Ester exerts amazing anti-aging power.

Six big advantages of vitamin C-Ester are:

1. It is less acidic than vitamin C.
2. It is fat soluble (vs. water soluble vitamin C).
3. It is easily absorbed into the skin.

4. When mixed into creams and lotions it is capable of keeping its potency for many years.
5. Vitamin C-Ester directly stimulates fibroblasts resulting in an increase in collagen and elastin in the dermis.
6. Vitamin C-Ester is less irritating to the skin. Hence, with inflamed skin in particular, vitamin C-Ester confers a huge benefit. Further, being lipid soluble is beneficial when it comes to fighting free radicals. Most of the free radical damage occurs around the lipid rich area of the cell membrane. Once absorbed, the lipid soluble vitamin C-Ester reaches high concentrations in this area exerting a powerful antioxidant effect. The lipid solubility of vitamin C-Ester allows it to penetrate the skin six times more efficiently than the water soluble 'regular' vitamin C.

Best Uses of Vitamin C-Ester

- Treatment of fine lines and wrinkles particularly on severely sun damaged skin. Vitamin C-Ester and any other skin ingredient that gets rid of fine lines and wrinkles should truly be considered 'anti-aging.'

- Sunburned, irritated or inflamed skin. Remember, through the blocking of inflammatory cells in the skin, vitamin C-Ester helps to calm the skin.

- Any area of skin that has lost collagen and is loose or saggy will show improvement through the use of vitamin C-Ester.

Vitamin E (Alpha-tocopherol)

Vitamin E is found throughout our body's membranes and tissues. The *alcohol based* alpha tocopherol penetrates the skin best (vs. alpha-tocopherol-*acetate*). Make sure you read the label and get alcohol based vitamin E. This anti-oxidant gem brings with it a cavalcade of benefits to the skin. It boosts collagen to reduce fine lines and wrinkles, helps fade age spots and has been shown to decrease sunburn damage and dryness if used prior to UV exposure. Offering antioxidant properties coupled with less swelling, redness, inflammation and wrinkles makes vitamin E one of my favorites.

Vitamin E can be taken in pill form and is also present in many foods. These include dark leafy greens, broccoli, almonds, sunflower seeds, avocado, squash and kiwifruit. Vitamin E is an antioxidant to remember when it comes to the maintenance of healthy skin. While vitamin E deficiency is not common, it can occur in certain conditions which affect the absorption of fats (i.e. Crohn's disease). Vitamin E has been shown to be of benefit in the prevention of diabetes, control of high blood sugar and treatment of some types of liver disease.

Vitamin E is found in normal sebum of the skin and is present in other membranes and tissues throughout the body. In addition to neutralizing free radicals it has a photo-protective effect. It absorbs the energy from UV rays while also reducing skin inflammation.

Vitamin E is also present to a greater degree in those who make more sebum. Remember, sebum comes from sebaceous (sweat) glands. Those who make more sebum tend to have oily skin with more vitamin E present. This is one of the reasons why those with oily skin tend to age more gracefully than those with dry skin. While vitamin E is normally only present in the epidermis, topical preparations of vitamin E can penetrate deeper into the dermal layers.

How Vitamin E Specifically Helps Your Skin:

1. Antioxidant – Vitamin E is what I consider one of several powerhouse antioxidants. Powerful neutralization of free radicals makes vitamin E a true anti-aging gem.

2. Photo-protection – It has been shown to decrease sunburn damage and skin dryness if used prior to UV exposure (especially UVB).

3. Topical vitamin E is able to penetrate into the dermis to boost collagen resulting in fewer fine lines and wrinkles.

4. Anti-inflammatory - Studies have demonstrated that vitamin E is particularly capable of reducing UV-induced skin inflammation (reduction of redness and swelling).

5. It is helpful in the reduction of excess skin pigment (age spots).

6. Wound healing – While many people may have used the liquid inside a vitamin E pill to apply to a wound to hasten healing, the data backing up the effectiveness of this option remains in question. The issue here appears to be the fact that the actual concentration of the vitamin E in this situation is too high. Hence, when mixed *with other skin healing ingredients* (i.e. at a lower concentration), evidence points to vitamin E offering a favorable outcome in the treatment of scars.

Green Tea

You don't need to go far to hear all the wonderful cures attributed to green tea. What it does to your skin is beautiful as well. Put simply, green tea has polyphenols. A really good type of polyphenol is *catechin,* which green tea is loaded with. Here is your antioxidant powerhouse. Through this it clears free radicals, prevents cell damage, repairs wrinkles and reduces inflammation. We know green tea is good for us. A 2005 study showed that women with moderate photo-aging responded equally well to topical vs. dietary green tea. There is also early evidence that green tea can block enzymes that break down collagen and elastin. We know that green tea in the form of cream or in the diet is helpful, to what degree is yet to be fully determined.

Resveratrol

Resveratrol was mentioned as far back as 1939 in a Japanese article after being isolated from a plant by Mr. Michio Takaoka. In 1963 it was isolated from the root of the Japanese knotweed plant.

Resveratrol comes from plants considered to be 'under stress.' It is a natural antioxidant best known today as a component of grapes and red wine. It is also found in blueberries, blackberries, raspberries, and nuts. Studies have demonstrated the ability of resveratrol to reduce inflammation in blood vessels while improving blood vessel function. In part, this is where the theory, 'A glass of wine is good for your heart' came from. Resveratrol does indeed contribute to the heart-healthy benefits of red wine.

When resveratrol is applied to the skin it protects against damaging UVB rays. Similar to green tea, resveratrol has polyphenols which are strong antioxidants. In a 2011 study, it was shown that resveratrol was exceptionally well suited for use on the skin due to these anti-oxidant properties. Other more limited studies have shown that its anti-inflammatory properties may indeed benefit acne as well. Clearly, there are better acne treatment options but resveratrol is one worth mentioning. Resveratrol has been gaining momentum in the skin care and anti-aging market primarily due to its powerful antioxidant effects.

Alpha Lipoic Acid

Alpha lipoic acid (ALA) is a sulfur-containing organic compound that can be taken both orally or applied topically (onto the skin). Alpha lipoic acid is a completely natural substance that is present in all of our cells. It is a very important ingredient in skin care. There are very few ingredients that bring so many anti-aging factors to the table. Alpha lipoic acid is a powerful antioxidant and so much more.

Alpha Lipoic Acid's Antioxidant Power:

Alpha lipoic acid (ALA) was discovered in 1951 as an essential ingredient in the mitochondria (powerhouse) of cells. Initial research showed that when additional alpha lipoic acid was made available to cells, it would quickly enter them and function as a powerful antioxidant. The beauty of ALA is that in addition to its own antioxidant power, it *enhances the antioxidant effects* of vitamins C and E. ALA has been called a 'universal' antioxidant due to the fact that it is *both lipid and water soluble*. This is important because it means that ALA is capable of exerting its antioxidant effects inside the cell, outside of the cell and between cells. Much of the free radical damage occurs on the surface of the cell (cell membrane) as well as between cells. ALA, being present throughout these areas is able to exert an antioxidant effect far superior to many others.

Fighting Inflammation

Skin inflammation causes skin damage and plays an important role in the formation of fine lines and wrinkles. In addition to the antioxidant effects, ALA prevents the production of *cytokines*; key substances the body releases in response to inflammation. ALA also blocks messenger cells associated with production of inflammatory enzymes. Blocking these enzymes is important as they can harm both the cell components as well as collagen. Therefore, through multiple pathways, ALA prevents and clears inflammation while preventing collagen breakdown.

Boosting Metabolism

Alpha Lipoic Acid (ALA) has the ability to affect the metabolism of the cell as well. ALA is normally found in the mitochondria of the cell (the cells powerhouse that determines the metabolic rate of the cell). ALA gives a boost to the metabolic rate of the cell which is important in anti-aging. Through improvements in the energy levels of the cell, ALA helps the cell more quickly absorb nutrients, remove waste and repair damage.

Protection of Collagen

Sugar (glucose) is necessary for our cells to stay alive and function normally. However, excess sugar interacts with collagen unfavorably. Collagen is a protein and when sugar attaches to it (a process known as *glycosylation*) cross-linking occurs. This results in collagen that is stiff, inelastic and un-flexible. When collagen is less flexible, so is the skin; it is less supple and smooth and more apt to form wrinkles. Here ALA comes to the rescue once again. Through prevention of collagen glycosylation, ALA has the ability to keep the sugar molecules from attaching to collagen thereby keeping the collagen fibers smooth and elastic.

Alpha Lipoic Acid Uses

Alpha lipoic acid's antioxidant and anti-aging effects help to improve skin texture and tone. This improves fine lines and wrinkles. Puffiness under the eyes or enlarged pores will improve with ALA treatment. I have found that the use of ALA seems to show the greatest improvement in those with a very dull complexion. The anti-inflammatory effects of ALA have been shown to be beneficial in the treatment of different causes of skin inflammation including eczema and rosacea.

Lycopene

Lycopene is a compound found in plants. It is involved with photosynthesis and helps to protect plants from constant exposure to UV rays. It gives many plants their vibrant red colors. Lycopene is found primarily in red fruits and vegetables. It can be taken orally or applied topically. Unlike alpha lipoic acid, the body does not have or make lycopene.

There are three ways that lycopene is beneficial to the skin. It is a powerful antioxidant, many times more potent than vitamin E. It has been shown to be beneficial in the formation of collagen and, while lycopene is not sunblock it does confer some UV protective effects as well.

Kojic acid

A by-product of the fermentation process of making sake (Japanese rice wine), kojic acid is a powerful antioxidant as well as an inhibitor of melanin production. Hence, in addition to clearing free radicals, it helps fade age spots, freckles and melasma. While I feel the kojic acid benefits are many, it is fairly unstable when mixed into cosmetic skin preparations. Upon exposure to sunlight it can lose its efficacy and change color. Kojic *dipalmitate* is an alternative used in many preparations as a substitute for regular kojic acid. The research does not fully support that this *dipalmitate* version is as powerful. I include kojic acid here as it clearly is a powerful antioxidant; however other antioxidants such as the ACE vitamins, in my experience, are preferable.

Any discussion of skin care and anti-aging is incomplete without mention of antioxidants. Free radicals are damaging to our bodies and our skin. When it comes to what we place onto our skin, every day we need antioxidant help. The use of these ingredients needs to be part of your daily routine. My favorites are vitamins A, C, E as well as alpha lipoic acid and resveratrol. Antioxidant = Anti-Aging. Next we discuss some other powerful anti-aging weapons for our skin.

Anti-Aging Winners

Dimethylaminoethanol (DMAE)

DMAE has been available in Europe for over 30 years as an oral supplement, known for its favorable effects on mental alertness. However, products such as ginkgo biloba and coenzyme Q10 have shown greater benefit in this regard. As a skin care ingredient, DMAE stabilizes membranes while exerting a powerful anti-inflammatory effect. It is a precursor to acetylcholine, a neurotransmitter crucial to contraction of muscles, including muscles of the face. Through improving muscle tone in the face, DMAE can prevent sagging and drooping of the overlying tissues.

When you think of the premise behind many medical aesthetic treatments, it is clear that wrinkles and sagging skin can be caused by several factors. In broad terms, this means loss of the supporting architecture of the skin; collagen and elastin. Hence, improvements in the amount and quality of collagen and elastin improve the skin's supporting architecture. Along these same lines, improved muscle tone beneath the dermis will strengthen and support the skin surface above.

This may seem contrary to the discussion of Botox, whereby the muscles themselves are temporarily paralyzed. On one hand, paralysis of the muscle brings a youthful appearance. In another, improved muscle tone results in the same. The important point here is that it's the repeated *contraction* of the muscle that results in wrinkles, not *tone*. Tone has nothing to do with muscle movement.

In regard to skin preparations, DMAE may come as a cream, serum or lotion and its application provides both short and long term benefits. In fact, studies of those using this ingredient for periods of 6 months to a year show that the improvements to skin smoothness and tone continue to occur. DMAE has an immediate effect *and* an additive effect.

DMAE Results

Results of topical use of DMAE include:

1. Fewer fine lines
2. Improved firmness
3. A 'lifting' effect
4. Improved radiance

I recommend using a pea sized drop of DMAE lotion spread over each side of the face paying particular attention to the naso-labial fold area, around the eye, the forehead and the chin, neck and décolletage area. Essentially any area of the face or neck can show improvement through the use of DMAE-containing topical preparations. Additionally, in many cases the skin appears more radiant with improvements of uneven skin tone.

Ceramides

The top layer of the epidermis is the stratum corneum. Ceramides make up 50% of this layer. Ceramides combine with cholesterol and saturated fatty acids, forming a layer that effectively prevents water loss. Hydrated skin is happy skin. It is important to drink plenty of fluids (four to five 16 ounce glasses/day) as well as keep healthy levels of these components in the stratum corneum. The composition of this upper layer of the epidermis is:

- 50% ceramides
- 25% cholesterol
- 15% free fatty acids

Note: In the face, the stratum corneum is 15-20 cell layers thick (average).

Additionally, the stratum corneum serves as a strong barrier against the entry of microorganisms. With age there is a steady decline in the ceramide and cholesterol present in the stratum corneum. This makes the skin more prone to dryness and the penetration of different environmental irritants including bacteria. The thickness of the stratum corneum differs depending on the area of the body it covers. It is thicker on the hands, feet, knees and elbows.

One of the best ways to keep this skin layer functioning well is to apply skin care products containing ceramides directly onto the skin surface. Products with a rich supply of ceramides both strengthen and refresh the skin surface, making it moist and more resistant to the external environment.

Ceramides in skin care products either come from plants or are synthetic. Both forms have been studied and neither has been proven to work significantly better than the other. Of the nine types of ceramides identified, nearly every type can be found in different skin care products. Typically they are present in moisturizers but are also in serums or lotions.

Ceramide Names Seen in Skin Care:

1. Ceramide AP
2. Ceramide EOP
3. Ceramide NG
4. Ceramide NP
5. Ceramide NS
6. Sphingosine
7. Phytosphingosine

Moisture is very important to your skin. Ceramides are a vital ingredient to consider in your skin care regimen. They protect the top skin layer while holding in precious moisture. Those with dry skin do particularly well through the use skin care products with ceramides.

Peptides

Peptides have become popular in recent years due to the manner in which they improve the skin at a cellular level. This means that they are able to penetrate the skin surface and enter into the individual cells. Peptides can reduce fine lines and wrinkles, shrink pore size, improve the skin color and texture while improving skin tightness. To a large extent the skin's appearance is based on the quality and quantity of the architecture supporting it. Here again we are talking about *collagen*. Young people have more collagen. This is a primary reason why they have fewer wrinkles. They have better architecture supporting the skin surface. With age we lose collagen along with the firmness, tightness and elasticity of the skin.

Collagen is a protein. There have been 28 types of collagen identified. 90% of the body's collagen (including that in the skin) is Type I. The body manufactures collagen through a complex biochemical process. However, like all else in medicine and skin care it can be explained rather simply. Think of it like this:

1. Protein (collagen) can be made in a couple of ways. One way is through the stringing together of amino acids.
2. When a protein is broken down, *peptides* are formed. These are 3-8 amino acid segments which can thereby *re-combine* with other amino acids to form protein.
3. Peptides therefore, serve as an essential building block of protein (collagen). This is why you pay so much for them in the form of serums or creams. Put very simply, peptides help your skin make more collagen.

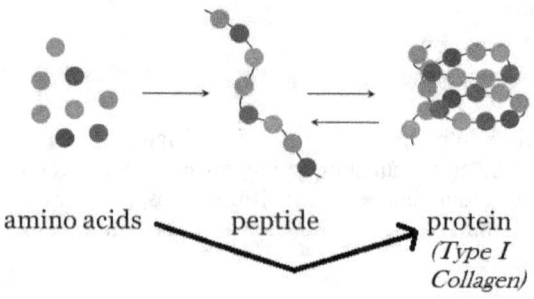

amino acids   peptide   protein
(Type I Collagen)

There are three types of peptides in the skin care and anti-aging market. Certain types of peptides are better at sending signals to the skin to make more collagen. Remember, it is collagen in the dermis that helps support the upper skin layer (epidermis). Regardless of what you do to the surface of your skin, you will never achieve enough tightness and elasticity if you don't gain more collagen.

Three Ways Peptides Help:

1.   They act as a signal to make more collagen.

As noted, when protein is broken down, peptides are formed. These peptides can combine with amino acids to form more protein. The fact that peptides are present, however, serves as a _signal_ that collagen has been broken down and needs to be replaced. Therefore, more peptides equate to a stronger signal for your body (skin) to make more protein (collagen).

Applying peptides directly to your skin thereby tricks your skin into making more collagen. The most popular 'signal peptide' seen in cosmetics is Palmitoyl Pentapeptide (Matrixyl). This can be found in many expensive and not-so-expensive formulations. Some examples include Strivectin NIA-114 and Oil of Olay Regenerist.

2.   They can deliver copper to your skin.

Because peptides are small, they can penetrate the skin's protective barriers to get into the deeper layers. When copper is attached to a peptide, the copper can be transported deeply into the skin as well. Research has demonstrated that copper is an effective agent in skin healing. For this reason it has been used for many years to treat chronic wounds. Copper peptides promote collagen production and act as antioxidants. They are needed for natural healing and regeneration of your skin. Copper peptides also help to remove damaged collagen.

3.   _Neuro_peptides may act like Botox.

Neuropeptides are peptides that play a role in nerve cell communication. Botox binds with facial nerves to ultimately prevent contraction of facial muscles. A neuropeptide known as **_argireline_** may block the release of neurotransmitters from nerves. In theory, if absorbed all the way to the level of the nerve and muscle, it could block contraction of the muscle leading to smoother skin and fewer wrinkles, much like Botox.

This is an area of great excitement in the world of medical aesthetics. One of the first neuropeptide creams by Dr. Perricone was touted to reduce wrinkles and make the skin smooth similar to Botox. This indeed worked, however not to the level of what is seen with Botox injections. This preparation has now been followed by many other neuropeptides as well as other 'topical' neurotoxins including bee and snake venom. These products claim to give similar results to Botox.

I would recommend you exercise caution in this area. I have no doubt that this sphere of medical aesthetics is on the verge of a huge change. Botox has been on top for a very long time. I would predict a neuropeptide replacement for Botox in the next three to five years. However, this preparation, if topical, would need to reach the level of the nerve and give a similar effect to that of Botox. While Botox allergies are essentially non-existent, allergies to these topical 'toxin' treatments are far more common. The day however is approaching when a "topical Botox" will be commonplace.

My Take on Peptides:

Peptides need to come in a preparation that affords adequate skin absorption. If they are incorporated into a heavy cream that is applied to the skin, there is little chance the peptides are going to do much other than sit on the skin surface. They also do not need to be extremely expensive. I am a proponent of the use of 'signal' peptides as well as copper peptides. These help your skin with the formation of collagen, bring antioxidant properties and aid in skin healing. Remember, your skin is a live, active organ. It is continually renewing itself. In regard to neuropeptides, it is my opinion that receiving a Botox treatment is the safest and most effective option for a reduction of wrinkles due to blocked nerve innervation. In this situation you are assured the nerve will be blocked and this has been scientifically proven again and again, which is not the case *today* with neuropeptides.

On the flip side, I am certain that more research and clinical studies are forthcoming to prove neuropeptides can do just what Botox can. What is necessary is the medium (cream or serum) used must be able to penetrate to the level of the nerve and muscle. Botox is the #1 of all medical aesthetic procedures ... but nobody stays on top forever.

Alpha and Beta Hydroxy Acids

Alpha and Beta hydroxy acids continue to be popular in the skin care world due to the many ways they help to improve the appearance of the skin. Alpha and Beta hydroxy acids are used for anti-aging, reversal of sun damage and treatment of acne. The primary difference in the uses of these two types of acids is related to their solubility (what they dissolve in). Alpha hydroxy acids are soluble in water (or water soluble) while beta hydroxy acids are soluble in oil (or lipid soluble). These differences dictate which one to choose to treat certain skin conditions.

Alpha Hydroxy Acids (AHAs)

Commonly used alpha hydroxy acids include glycolic (from sugar cane), lactic (from milk), malic (from apples), citric (from citrus fruit), and tartaric (from grape wine). Glycolic acid is the smallest molecule thus allowing for the deepest skin penetration. Hence glycolic acid is the AHA used most widely.

AHAs work in several ways to improve the appearance of the skin. Their most important role is skin exfoliation. The term 'exfoliation' is defined as *removal of the surface*. Once the skin cells have died they are sloughed to the outer skin surface (the stratum corneum). The AHAs clear away the outermost dead skin cells from the surface. Through exfoliation, AHAs accomplish two things. First, removal of the outer dead cells gives the skin a healthy glow. Second, the actual process of exfoliation speeds up the formation of new cells at the base of the epidermis (at the stratum basale). Therefore, you have now hastened the process of formation of new cells.

Since AHAs (particularly glycolic acid) penetrate deeply, they also stimulate the growth of deeper supporting components of the skin (collagen and elastin). Glycolic, lactic and citric acids work particularly well at increasing collagen and skin thickness. Continued use of these AHAs will therefore help to 'fill in' wrinkles making the skin smoother and more even. Skin care ingredients that promote exfoliation and improved cell turnover (such as retinol) will also help improve unwanted pigment. This characteristic of AHAs makes them effective in reducing unwanted or uneven skin pigment as well. With AHAs we have new vibrant skin surface with a boost of the 'architecture' supporting it.

Beta Hydroxy Acids (BHA)

Salicylic acid is the primary beta hydroxy acid (BHA) used in skin care. Salicylic acid is a derivative of aspirin giving it anti-inflammatory properties. Salicylic acid also brings anti-irritant, anti-redness, and anti-microbial properties. Unlike AHAs, BHAs are soluble in oil (lipid), resulting in deep penetration into the sebum-containing pore. Thus, BHAs clear sebum and dead skin cells built up inside the pore. This makes BHAs an excellent choice for use on oily skin or acne-prone skin (with blackheads/whiteheads). Deep penetration into the pore and clearing of sebum and dead skin cells is what it does best. BHAs are most effective at lower concentrations (around 2%). Like AHA, the use of BHA has been shown to reduce the presence of wrinkles and pigment changes caused by sun damage. With BHA the results come but may take up to six months.

Similarities

AHAs and BHAs both do a beautiful job of exfoliating the skin (clearing away dead skin cells). AHAs can be more irritating and it is recommended to start slowly if you have never used them before. I recommend beginning with an every-other-day schedule and change accordingly depending on skin irritation. BHAs are effective at lower concentrations and tend to be preferred by dermatologists as they are less irritating.

Both AHAs and BHAs, through clearing dead skin cells and increasing cell turnover, can improve the thickness of the skin, the skins barrier properties as well as stimulate growth of collagen and elastin in the dermis. Regardless, when using AHAs or BHAs you need to wear sun block. These acids, through lowering the skin PH, clearing away dead skin cells and removing protective oils, make your skin up to 50 % more likely to burn. Make certain to use sun block to protect against both UVA and UVB rays when using products containing alpha or beta hydroxy acids.

Niacinamide

Niacin (Vitamin B3) is a water soluble vitamin that combines with amino acids to produce niacinamide (also referred to as nicotinamide and nicotinic amide). Most people receive enough of this essential vitamin from their daily diet through consumption of fish, fortified breads, nuts and multivitamins. Niacinamide, while a necessary daily vitamin, works beautifully if applied to the skin.

Niacinamide has the ability to help cells communicate with one another. It is involved with enzymatic reactions that give it an antioxidant quality. It also repairs damage to cells, including repair to the cell DNA. It improves the barrier function of the skin while stimulating the microcirculation in the dermis. The circulation to the skin although vitally important … is frequently forgotten.

There is no direct blood supply to the epidermis. It all comes through small vessels just below the epidermis in the dermal layer. Circulation is vital to the skin. As the dermal circulation improves, more nutrients and oxygen are delivered to the skin and waste products are thoroughly and efficiently removed. Therefore, without a brisk circulation the skin suffers. Exercise improves circulation to the skin while a diet high in antioxidants delivers powerful anti-aging factors. These elements are of utmost importance in overall skin health.

In addition to improved circulation, niacinamide also increases ceramide and free fatty acid levels in the skin. This is helpful to dry skin and skin with unwanted or uneven pigment. It also brings anti-inflammatory properties that have a calming effect on the skin.

Look for daily skin care products containing niacinamide. It is a true member of your Winning Skin arsenal.

Skin Benefits of Niacinamide:

1. Improved barrier function of the epidermis
2. Reduction of brown spots

3. Improvement of uneven skin texture
4. Reduction of fine lines and wrinkles
5. Reduction of inflammation and redness
6. Improved circulation to the dermis (and epidermis)
7. Reduction of sebum production
8. It helps rosacea – Niacinamide has been shown to enhance the skin's barrier function in rosacea patients, resulting in a diminished reaction to irritants. One study demonstrated that treatment with niacinamide resulted in clinical improvement in 26 out of 34 subjects with mild to moderate rosacea.
9. It helps acne - In a study published in the International Journal of Dermatology, 4% niacinamide gel was compared to 1% clindamycin gel (a topical antibiotic) in patients with moderate inflammatory acne. After 8 weeks, 82% of patients treated with niacinamide and 68% of those treated with clindamycin were considered improved.
10. Improvement of dry skin – Topical niacinamide moisturizers were shown to be helpful in the treatment of those suffering from certain types of dry skin such as atopic dermatitis.

As a group, people spend millions of dollars on anti-aging skin care. Niacinamide offers many benefits at a fraction of the cost. A 2008 study in the Journal of Dermatology showed a significant improvement in crow's feet wrinkles after being treated with topical niacinamide for 8 weeks. With all the benefits seen it is important to note that side effects are quite rare with niacinamide and are limited to minimal skin irritation in a very small percentage of users.

Hydroquinone

Hydroquinone is arguably the most effective skin lightening cream available today. It is primarily used to treat age spots (liver spots), melasma, freckles, acne scars or other types of skin discolorations. Hydroquinone has been around a long time. It works very well and is a go-to ingredient for unwanted pigment.

How Hydroquinone Works:

The skin has pigment cells called melanocytes. Inside melanocytes are melanosomes which contain melanin. Melanin is what gives our skin its pigment. Tyrosinase is an enzyme needed to make melanin. UVA/UVB ray exposure increases the production of melanin, thus causing our skin to become tan. Sunbathers in search of a deep dark tan are simply attempting to acquire more melanin in the skin's pigment cells. When hydroquinone is applied to the skin *the tyrosinase enzyme becomes blocked.* With tyrosinase not functioning normally, less melanin is produced. The end result is lighter skin. With the use of hydroquinone many of the visible areas of unwanted pigment will fade, but it goes a step further. Studies have shown that the use of hydroquinone is capable of even reducing pigment that has not yet reached the skin surface (i.e. not visible yet).

The Opposite of UV rays:

Hydroquinone's action on our skin is essentially the opposite of what UV rays do. Instead of more melanin being produced, the melanin production is blocked. The result is lighter skin and fading of dark (hyper-pigmented) spots. It comes as no surprise that those using hydroquinone are very prone to damaging sun rays. Blocking melanin production makes it very easy to suffer sunburn. Our defense against the sun (melanin) is now far less available.

Therefore, when using hydroquinone one should stay out of the sun or at minimum use a sun block with SPF 50 vs. UVA/UVB rays. Hydroquinone is commonly referred to as a 'bleaching cream.' While it does make the skin lighter, it is important to understand that it is not from *actual bleaching* of the skin, rather from the reduction of the skin's *production* of melanin.

Hydroquinone Preparations:

Depending on which country you reside, different strengths of hydroquinone are available over the counter (OTC). In the US, preparations of up to 2% are available OTC; higher percentages require a visit to the doctor for a prescription. With the use of hydroquinone 2% many people are lulled into thinking that since it is OTC, it is safe. This is strong medicine and needs to be used cautiously. The reason it is so popular is that it works well; however, while I have seen excellent results with the use of hydroquinone, I have also seen many side effects. Careless use of hydroquinone may result in skin irritation and sunburn.

Safety and Side Effects:

As noted, hydroquinone reduces the amount of melanin produced in skin cells. Melanin is essential to protecting your skin from UVA/UVB rays. With the lower defense your skin has against the sun, you need to take extra precautions to compensate for these lowered defenses. Many hydroquinone preparations come with sun block. If not, you need to make sure you are adding it when using hydroquinone.

Anyone using a product containing hydroquinone for the first time should perform a skin test. Simply apply a small amount of the cream to a quarter-sized area of unbroken skin (the forearm is a good area). Check the area for 24 hours to determine if you are allergic. If the skin becomes puffy, red or extremely itchy, discontinue use and, if severe, contact your doctor. Mild itching is normal, and in this case, the treatment may be applied to the desired area. If the skin becomes cracked, blistered or unwanted skin changes occur you should cleanse the area and discontinue use. If you suffer from asthma or skin conditions including eczema or psoriasis, speak to your doctor before starting hydroquinone. It should not be used in pregnant or nursing women. Finally, make sure you only use it on your skin and keep it out of your nose and eyes.

The Good News:

The discussion of beauty-improving skin care ingredients is incomplete without a discussion of hydroquinone. While it is important to discuss potential side effects and the need to exercise caution with its use, the fact is that most every person who wants to clear away unwanted pigmented does exceptionally well through the use of hydroquinone. I recommend its use twice daily for 6-8 weeks for optimal results. Once you have seen results, the best way to preserve your clearer skin is to make sure you keep using sun block.

Beauty Oils

Many people are hesitant to try essential oils or 'beauty oils' due to concerns they have in regard to clogging pores, allergies or simply discomfort on the skin. The beauty industry and skin care world has advanced far beyond the simple mineral oil based products of the 1970s. Today we are indeed fortunate to have so many beauty oil options when it comes to skin care. A wide range of skin conditions including excess pigment, dry skin, oily skin and sensitive skin may be effectively treated through the use of oils. Further, many bring anti-aging qualities and even help conditions like rosacea and acne. Be careful though, some oils block pores and these are the ones to steer clear of with acne prone skin.

The majority of people think of oils in terms to how they can help keep the skin moist. When discussing moisturizers, it is important to understand and reiterate three important definitions:

(A review of) Humectants, Occulsives and Emollients

A Humectant such as glycerin or hyaluronic acid *attracts and retains* moisture in your skin.

An Occlusive works by forming a thin film on the surface of the skin to *prevent loss* of moisture.

An Emollient helps to make the external skin layers more *soft and supple*. In doing so, skin hydration is improved and evaporation reduced.

Oils fall into the ***occlusive and emollient*** categories. It would make sense that those that were more 'occlusive' would be more prone to blocking pores. Hyaluronic acid as a humectant it does a beautiful job of drawing moisture into your skin. It's like a moisture magnet. Oils are not moisture magnets, they are moisture *traps*. They prevent the moisture from leaving. Your skin has a certain percentage of water whether or not you are using a humectant like hyaluronic acid. Using a humectant will add to the moisture already present in your skin. Using a beauty oil will help trap that moisture in. The layering of ingredients is important here. If you are using a moisturizer it should be put on *before* the beauty oil. Simply put, the humectant (hyaluronic acid) attracts water, and the oil helps to keep it there.

Coconut Oil (anti-aging, antioxidant)

I am a fan of skin care that smells good, is simple to use and gives results. Coconut oil does just that. The only drawback is its higher tendency to block pores than other oils. There are many reasons why coconut oil has become so popular. The fact that is smells like a day at the beach has nothing to do with why it is helpful to your skin. There are straightforward reasons why it helps and others which have been a source of some controversy.

Coconut Oil Contains Lauric Acid

Coconut oil has some important ingredients; medium chain fatty acids and triglycerides. These do an excellent job of keeping moisture in the skin where it belongs. Hydrated skin is happy and beautiful skin. Lauric acid is one of the important fatty acids in coconut oil (also present in palm kernel oil). Lauric acid helps to moisturize the skin but it goes a step further. It brings anti-bacterial properties which some experts argue is helpful in treating acne. The premise is that lauric acid fuses to the membrane of the bacteria thereby preventing it from spreading. I agree that coconut oil has anti-bacterial qualities. The problem is that coconut oil is very *comedogenic.*

Comedogenesis is defined as, "tendency to clog pores especially by the formation of blackheads."

Hence, if a product is more comedogenic, it is prone to either cause acne or worsen it if present. As you can see from the following table, coconut oil is one of the most comedogenic beauty oils.

Those who treat acne and those that suffer from it realize that two primary goals are to 1) get rid of dead skin cells and 2) keep pores clear. There are more effective ways to clear bacteria from the skin of those suffering from acne. Benzoyl peroxide, for instance, is an antibacterial agent that gets inside the pore and helps to kill bacteria while also reducing inflammation. Now, if you do not suffer from acne, coconut oil and its lauric acid do a beautiful job of moisturizing and conditioning the skin. If you have acne and enjoy the moisturizing effects of beauty oils, tea tree oil is a far better option.

COMEDOGENESIS

Non-Comedogenic	Mildly Comedogenic	Moderately Comedogenic	Most Comedogenic
Argan Oil	Calendula Oil	Almond Oil	Cocoa Butter
Marula Oil	Jojoba Oil *	Apricot Oil	**Coconut Oil**
Tea Tree Oil *	Chamomile Oil	Avocado Oil	Corn Oil
Hemp Seed Oil	Emu Oil	Olive Oil	Flaxseed Oil
Safflower Oil	Grape Seed Oil	Peanut Oil	Mink Oil
Sunflower Oil	Pomegranate Oil	Primrose Oil	Soybean Oil
Mineral Oil	Rosehip Oil	Sesame Oil	Wheat Germ Oil

Better for acne – Tea Tree Oil and Jojoba Oil

Coconut Oil Contains Vitamin E

With vitamin E (alpha-tocopherol) present, coconut oil brings collagen boosting and anti-inflammatory qualities. Thus, coconut oil brings anti-aging qualities to the table in helping to reduce fine lines and wrinkles.

Coconut Oil is an Antioxidant

Its antioxidant properties neutralize free radicals, stimulate collagen production, repair cells and help to fade redness.

Coconut Oil Has an SPF of 8

Coconut oil is able to block harmful UVA and UVB rays. Remember if you can stay in the sun 15 minutes before burning, an SPF of 8 allows you to say out 8 times longer (or 2 hours). In addition to the SPF factor, it also has a natural anti-inflammatory property which can help to soothe irritated skin.

Other Coconut Oil Uses:

1. Lip balm – Your lips are exposed to the same UVA/UVB rays as the rest of your face. Some people's lips get dry and chapped in the low-humidity winter months while others experience this year round. Coconut oil does a great job as a lip moisturizer and protector.

2. Body Oil – Many suffer from dry areas of the skin including hands, feet and heels, knees or elbows. Coconut oil is very helpful in moisturizing these dry and irritated areas. Argan oil is another excellent body oil choice.

3. Under eye cream – There are certainly more powerful eye creams available than coconut oil. However, it is an option to consider for fine lines and wrinkles under and around the eyes. It's not Botox, but it is helpful, particularly with dry skin.

4. Exfoliant – using equal parts of sea salt and coconut oil, this is an option for a home-made exfoliant.

5. Shaving 'lotion' – Many women swear by the use of coconut oil for shaving their legs. It moisturizes and leaves legs smooth and soft. Men with sensitive skin find that coconut oil is a viable shaving lotion option as well.

Argan Oil - (anti-aging, antioxidant, melanin inhibitor)

Argan Oil contains vitamins A and E (antioxidants) and essential fatty acids. This beauty oil has become very popular in recent years, and for good reason. Clients of mine have seen amazing results literally all over their body using this oil (face, hands, feet, elbows and hair). It doesn't clog pores, does a beautiful job maintaining hydration and is described by many as feeling 'light' on the skin. Unlike other antioxidants, argan oil remains very stable when exposed to UV rays. It terms of antioxidant power, it is one of the very best. The Journal of Evidence Based Complementary and Alternative Medicine described Argan oil as "an effective melanin biosynthesis inhibitor." It certainly is not a first choice as far as reduction of pigment but it does have the ability to reduce it more so than other beauty oils.

Marula Oil - (anti-aging, skin discolorations, inflammation)

Marula oil is a beauty oil gem. It was originally harvested in South Africa from the nut inside the marula fruit. It has 60% more antioxidant power than argan oil. It contains vitamin E, essential amino and fatty acids (omega 6 and 9). It also contains loads of vitamin C. Remember, vitamin C in addition to its antioxidant properties, stimulates collagen, reduces inflammation and fades skin discolorations. Marula oil's composition makes it far less likely to irritate the skin than other beauty oils. It is non-comedogenic which makes it an excellent choice for acne-prone skin.

Rosehip Oil (anti-aging, skin discolorations)

Rosehip oil contains essential fatty acids, lots of vitamin C and E (antioxidants) and B-carotene (Pro-Vitamin A). In addition to trapping moisture, rosehip oil packs a true anti-aging punch through the fading of dark spots and reduction of fine lines and minor scars. Rosehip oil recently received a slew of positive press and increased sales following its support by Gwyneth Paltrow and the Duchess of Cambridge.

Jojoba Oil – (anti-inflammatory, acne, dry skin, sensitive skin)

With vitamins E and B-complex, copper and zinc, jojoba oil brings with it powerful skin benefits. It closely resembles human sebum (the substance made by sebaceous glands). It may not make sense that you would put something onto your skin that mimics pore-blocking sebum. With jojoba oil it makes perfect sense. Jojoba oil has the paradoxical effect of tricking your skin into 'thinking' there is more than enough sebum present. Hence, the skin actually produces *less* sebum. Jojoba oil helps clear the skin and open clogged pores. It brings antibacterial properties vs. acne bacteria (*proprionibacterium acnes*). Jojoba oil very non-allergenic and is helpful particularly with dry or sensitive skin types.

Olive Oil – (very dry skin, anti-aging)

When buying olive oil one should look for extra virgin olive oil. Fatty acids, squalene and polyphenols (which help blood flow and skin oxygenation) are key ingredients. Olive oil is a good choice for its anti-aging and moisture retaining effects particularly in those with very dry skin.

Grapeseed Oil (oily skin, acne, anti-inflammatory)

Grapeseed oil helps to regulate your skin's normal oil production making it an excellent choice for oily skin. It contains amino acids and plenty of vitamin C and all the antioxidant power that comes with it. Grapeseed oil is light, odorless, anti-inflammatory and mildly astringent (i.e. constricts pores).

Pomegranate Oil – (anti-aging, anti-inflammatory)

Rich in vitamins A, C, E (antioxidant powerhouse vitamins), pomegranate oil brings antioxidant, anti-inflammatory and antimicrobial properties. The vitamin C helps to fade dark spots while stimulating fibroblasts to make more collagen and elastin.

Sunflower Seed Oil (anti-aging, dry skin)

Sunflower oil has light consistency that is similar to human sebum. It can be used as a substitute for coconut oil in those with acne-prone skin. Sunflower seed oil is rich in vitamins that improve the health and radiance of your skin, including vitamins A, D and E. In addition, it contains essential fatty acids and carotenoids that help prevent skin cancer. Sunflower seed oil nourishes and moisturizes many skin types. With oily skin types there are better options such as grapeseed oil.

Chamomile Oil (anti-inflammatory, sensitive skin, eczema, rosacea)

Chamomile tea has been known for ages for its calming effects so it comes as no surprise that chamomile oil is calming to the skin as well. Chamomile oil's strong anti-inflammatory properties have been shown to be beneficial in conditions such as eczema and rosacea. It is also well suited for those with sensitive skin.

Tea Tree Oil (acne, anti-inflammatory)

25 years ago the Medical Journal of Australia showed that 5% tea tree oil was as effective as 5% benzoyl peroxide in a study of 124 patients with inflammatory acne. Tea tree oil worked more slowly to reduce open and closed comedones, but also caused fewer side effects than benzoyl peroxide. It has also been shown to have activity against the fungus present in skin and nail infections. Tea tree oil is non-comedogenic and beneficial in the treatment of mild to moderate inflammatory acne.

Wheat Germ Oil (dry skin, antioxidant, anti-inflammatory)

Wheat germ oil is excellent for dry and irritated skin. It is an excellent moisturizer with loads of vitamin E, making it a powerful antioxidant as well. This oil also brings strong anti-inflammatory properties. Its high content of vitamin E means it helps vitamin C work more effectively. It can also be used to help dry and cracked elbows, heels and feet. Stay away from this oil with acne-prone skin.

Beauty Oil Allergies

I noted earlier that many people are fearful to try beauty oils due to potential skin allergies. Certain oils like avocado oil and almond oil do bring more potential for allergies than the others. Before you cover your face or body with any of these oils it is strongly recommended that you test a small quarter-sized area on your forearm to see if you are potentially allergic. While allergies to oils are not common, they are present.

Grape Seed Extract

As a quick review of how we are to attain the best anti-aging results.

We need to:

1. Improve the architecture supporting the epidermis (collagen and elastin).
2. Improve the health of the epidermis.
3. Prevent damage to these layers.

This is accomplished via:

1. Helping to clear (or prevent) free radicals through the use of antioxidants (topical and dietary), UV protection and reduction of inflammation.
2. Improvement of epidermal cell turnover (i.e. exfoliation).
3. Products or procedures that boost collagen and elastin.

There are hundreds of ways to accomplish what I have listed above. Visit me at ClearSkinMD.net. Here you can ask me and our expert staff questions directly. For example, if you want to find out if a product you are considering has the ingredients necessary to accomplish your goal, we are pleased to help.

Grape seed extract is made from the ground seeds of red wine grapes. The molecular size of the liquid extract from these seeds allows for excellent absorption into the skin.

A 2014 study of the Global Journal of Health Science showed the topical use of grape seed extract triggered the release of growth factors, proliferation of healthy epidermal skin layers along with anti-inflammatory and anti-microbial properties. The use of grape seed extract made a skin wound heal fully in 8 days vs. 14 days in the placebo group. Your skin loves grape seed extract.

What Grape Seed Extract Contains:

1. Oligomeric Procyanidins (OPCs)

These OPCs exert a strong anti-oxidant effect when applied to the skin. I have mentioned that vitamin E is one of my favorite vitamins, in part, due to its antioxidant power. According to a report from the Food and Research Center in Guelph, Canada, OPCs in grape seed extract were shown to contain 20 times the antioxidant power of vitamin E and 50 times the antioxidant power of vitamin C. This is big-time antioxidant (and anti-aging) strength.

2. Resveratrol

This is a strong anti-oxidant with anti-inflammatory properties. Resveratrol has also been shown to have antibacterial and antifungal properties as well. Resveratrol stimulates proliferation of healthy epidermal skin cells and stimulates fibroblasts to make new collagen and elastin. Through resveratrol's powerful anti-oxidant properties, it prevents damage to the collagen and elastin matrix in the dermis.

3. Polyphenols

Studies have shown conclusively that application of polyphenols to the skin protects against UV rays while improving epidermal skin growth. Polyphenols have also been shown (when taken orally) to improve dermal blood flow and oxygen delivery to the skin, resulting in statistically significant improvements in skin texture and tone.

Grape seed extract is clearly a friend to your skin. It packs a powerful anti-oxidant punch along with anti-inflammatory, anti-bacterial, anti-fungal and wound healing properties.

Organic Skin Care

The term 'organic' always held a special meaning to me. In 1986 at The University of Wisconsin I studied organic chemistry. The "B+" I received may go down as one of my greatest achievements. Little did I know back then when I was studying day and night for this nightmarish course that the word 'organic' would become so popular in the 21st century. In 2013, organic skin care was an 8 billion dollar industry. By 2020 this will double to 16 billion. In terms of the overall skin care market, the 8% organic share of 2012 will grow to 12% by 2020.

Defining Organic

The general definition is: *relating to or denoting compounds containing carbon and chiefly of biologic origin.*

In regard to food or farming: *produced or involving production without the use of chemicals, fertilizers, pesticides or other artificial agents.*

The USDA National Organic Program (NOP) has a lengthy definition of 'organic' which essentially says farmers use no pesticides, antibiotics or fertilizers not government approved as organic. The NOP follows farmers and companies closely to make sure these guidelines are followed.

The FDA's Description of Organic

It is clear that the FDA (US Food and Drug Administration) has the intent of protecting the consumer. They closely monitor foods, beverages and most certainly medication. When it comes to skin care and cosmetics, the FDA's watchful eye is less focused. The skin is a sponge and may absorb up to 80% of what is applied to it, so why isn't organic skin care watched more closely?

According to FDA.gov:

Manufacturers are not required to register their cosmetic establishments or file their product formulations with the FDA.

In terms of organic skin care: The FDA doesn't really have a definition of "organic." They state:

An ingredient's source does not determine its safety. For example, many plants, whether or not they are organically grown, contain substances that may be toxic or allergenic."

This actually makes a lot of sense. Simply saying something is organic does not necessarily mean it is safe. Poison ivy is *organic*. That doesn't mean it is safe to rub all over our skin.

Organic skin care need not be difficult or confusing.

1. Read the ingredients remembering that the first item listed under active ingredients is what the product contains the most of. All ingredients are important here, but the top 1/3 of the list warrants special attention.

2. Emollients, humectants, emulsifiers, surfactants and preservatives have uses for the skin. This should give you some guidelines to follow in terms of what is considered organic and what should be avoided.

   - **Emollient**– Used to prevent drying. It makes the skin layers more soft and supple. Emollients have an ability to act as healing agents. Organic emollients include jojoba, avocado, rosehip, shea and cocoa.

   - **Humectants**– Attract and retain moisture. In doing so they keep the skin well hydrated. Organic humectants include natural phospholipids such as lecithin and panthenol (also known as pro-vitamin B-5).

   - **Emulsifiers**– hold ingredients together. Organic emulsifiers include carnauba, jojoba, quince, xanthan gum and rice bran.

- **Surfactants** – Dissolve oils and help to remove dirt. They are typically used with cleansers. Organic surfactants include castle soap, yucca extract, quillaja bark extract and soapwort.

- **Preservatives**– Preserve and extend the life of the product. Organic preservatives include tea tree oil, grapefruit seed extract and bitter orange extract.

What is 100% Organic?

Something that is labeled as "100% Organic" must contain only organically produced ingredients*

"Organic" labeling means at least 95% of the product has organically produced ingredients*

*excludes water and salt.

What to Avoid and Why

1. Isopropyl Alcohol (SD-40): A solvent that is drying and irritating. Will cause excessive skin dryness and stripping of protective oils. It is very drying to the skin.

2. FD and C Color Pigments: Animal studies have shown these synthetic colors may cause certain cancers.

3. Synthetic Fragrances: I prefer to stay away from heavy un-natural fragrances altogether and encourage my clients to do so as well. They tend to be both drying and irritating to the skin. Many people have allergies to synthetic fragrances.

4. Diethanolamine (DEA), Monoethanolamine (MEA) and Triethanolamine (TEA): Keep an eye out for these in skin care products. They are the precursors to nitrates and nitrosamines which are known to cause certain cancers.

5. <u>DMDM Hydantoin and Urea:</u>
   These preservatives release formaldehyde.

6. <u>Mineral Oil:</u> The early beauty oils were largely mineral oil based. It tends to be very heavy and uncomfortable on the skin particularly with sensitive or oily skin types. There are many better options available today. Though it is considered non-comedogenic, there are many better choices for those with acne-prone skin.

7. <u>PEG (poly-ethylene glycol) or PPG (poly propylene glycol):</u> These ingredients are potentially carcinogenic. They can alter or reduce the skin's natural moisture barrier

8. Others to stay away from:

   - Urea containing products
   - Propylene glycol and butylene glycol
   - Sodium lauryl sulfate
   - Aluminum
   - Toluene
   - PABA
   - Camphor
   - Formaldehyde

This is not an exhaustive list, however check your app store for a free app known as *"think dirty."* This allows you to scan the bar code of products to give you a clearer picture of the ingredients present.

Chapter Four

Exfoliation and Cell Turnover

Christie Brinkley remains one of the most photographed women in the world. She gained worldwide fame in the late 70s with three consecutive Sports Illustrated swimsuit issue covers. Men's Health and Allure Magazine named her the 'most attractive woman of all time' and she has appeared on the cover of over 500 magazines.

She was the prize of CoverGirl reigning as their queen for 25 years. She has always had a beautiful and radiant glow which appears to defy age. At the time of this writing she is 62 and looks absolutely amazing. If there is a fountain of youth, Christie has found it.

In many cases people are quick to say that celebrities have the best skin care, the best doctors and undergo procedure after procedure to retain a youthful appearance. This is certainly true in many cases. Christie has hit the 'genetics lottery' and has a personal dermatologist. That's both luck and luxury. However, not everyone with money and good genes looks as youthful and beautiful as Christie. She had to work at it too.

Importance of Exfoliation

When Christie was recently interviewed, she brought forth part of her skin care regimen present since her twenties. It made perfect sense to me. Christie, amongst other things, is a big fan of exfoliation.

Most men shave their face every day. Whether they realize it or not, this is exfoliation. That thin razor blade, along with removing hair, is slicing away dead skin cells. Christie read about this fact early in her career and has been exfoliating ever since. That's right, beautiful Christie has been exfoliating for 40 years. We will discuss many means to looking younger, feeling younger and aging gracefully. Regular exfoliation is of utmost importance to your anti-aging plan.

Exfoliation (eks-foh-lee-**ey**-shuh n) is defined in skin care as *removal of the surface*. Put bluntly, dead skin cells are not your friend. It doesn't matter if your skin is oily, dry, normal or sensitive. You need to regularly clear the upper layer of dead skin cells. When excess dead skin cells are present, your complexion is dull with more fine lines, wrinkles and blocked pores.

By exfoliating, you clear these skin-dulling cells from the top layer of the epidermis (stratum corneum). In doing so it prevents them from blocking your pores. This is *so important* because when pores are clogged with dead cells they look larger. If they are blocked long enough blackheads and whiteheads (acne) can result. Some people genetically have smaller pores, but anyone who exfoliates will have smaller pores and smoother skin.

The epidermis has five layers. The top skin layer is the stratum corneum. These are dead cells that lie atop the lower layers. The new cells come from the stratum basale and move upward until they reach the surface. I have mentioned the average life of a skin cell is 3-4 weeks. This is true more so in younger adults who have a rate of complete cell turnover of 24-28 days. As people age, cell turnover becomes sluggish. In those that are 60+ the rate of cell turnover is nearly twice as slow at 45-55 days. The dead skin cells on the surface do serve some protective function, however, more dead skin cells means more fine lines, wrinkles and a less vibrant complexion. Getting rid of excess dead skin cells on the surface stimulates the epidermis to make more 'new' cells from the stratum basale.

Therefore, exfoliation speeds up the entire process. This results in newer and fresher cells moving upward to the stratum corneum to replace the 'older' dead skin cells. This improves skin texture and results in smaller pores. People that exfoliate regularly are making huge strides toward clearer, smoother and more vibrant skin with smaller pores and fewer fine lines and wrinkles. In some cases it can even help to fade discolorations.

I separate exfoliation into two large groups; physical exfoliation and chemical exfoliation.

Physical Exfoliation

Physical exfoliation means you are using a cleanser or a product with beads, microbeads or powder with the goal of clearing away dead cells. In many cases the product is applied to the face in tandem with a mechanical pad that rotates in circles or vibrates as it is applied. Other people may simply put the exfoliant on a wash cloth, loofah or simply just let their fingers perform the same circular motion. Some people have gone to bypassing company products altogether and make their own exfoliants at home using ingredients like sugar, coffee, oatmeal, baking soda and sea salt. Even if you are applying a mild cleanser to your face with your fingers using a circular motion; this is exfoliation.

Here is my take on physical exfoliation:

First, loofahs tend to be a bit rough on the skin. I mention loofahs as many people use them and they can be drying to the skin. There are many better options. Second, if you are using a rotating or vibrating exfoliating brush let the pad to the work. Don't push so hard you can feel your teeth vibrating. In fact, don't push much at all! Better yet, use a soft washcloth. I prefer people use their fingers when exfoliating. Your fingers have nerve endings hence you can *feel* what you are doing. This is not to say I am against the use of a rotating pad or washcloth. The point to remember is you are removing a fine layer of dead cells with healthy and beautiful cells beneath. Scrubbing too hard is not going to give you better results and may just irritate your skin. You also have protective oils on the skin surface. Aggressively stripping all these oils away can leave your skin very dry. I tell people to imagine exfoliating a baby's face. With this image in mind you are less likely to be overly aggressive or over-scrub your skin surface.

There are many effective ways to physically exfoliate your skin. In fact there are many products out there that all say they will exfoliate your skin better than the next. Since I am a patient advocate at heart, it is important to review these exfoliating devices and draw some conclusions in regard to what works and what doesn't. Remember, in order to keep pores clear and open, we need to get rid of the dead skin cells that can clog them. Further, removal of these dead cells stimulates the skin's process of making new cells to take the place of the dead ones. Small and clear pores and a fresh vibrant surface is the goal.

A Review of Ten Exfoliating Devices

I want to be clear that there is nothing wrong with exfoliating with your fingertips. There are many exfoliating devices on the market and it is important to understand which you can trust. Let's begin with a discussion of how to use them. Devices either come with a rotating head or a vibrating (sonic) head.

Using Exfoliating Devices:

1. Refrain from repeating the same pattern when exfoliating your skin. Do not continually push 'up and out' toward your hairline. Mix it up.
2. Make sure you make an extra pass over the T-zone area. The forehead, brow, nose and chin make up an area of your face in a 'T' shape. It is important to make an extra pass over this area as it tends to be oilier than the rest of the face. *On average* this area has more sebaceous glands.

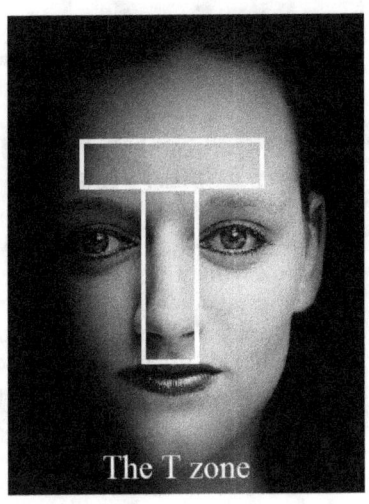

The T zone

3. Use the device once a day as see how your skin tolerates it. There is no set schedule *for everyone* for use of these devices. People use them anywhere from weekly to twice daily. I typically exfoliate every other day. That works for me. Find out what works for you. In my opinion, less is more.

4. Don't scrub. We are trying to gently exfoliate the upper layers of the epidermis. A common complaint, particularly of rotating exfoliating devices, is that they don't 'have enough power.' Remember, if you push *hard enough* any of these devices will lose power.

5. Start with a gentle cleanser. If your face tolerates that well, you may try more aggressive measures such as exfoliation products with beads, microbeads or powder aimed at helping to clear away dead cells.

6. Remember that if you are exfoliating too aggressively, your skin will become dry and irritated. This can result in the sebaceous glands in your face receiving a signal to make more oil. The goal should remain gentle exfoliation.

Of the ten devices reviewed to aid you with your physical exfoliation goal, five were rotating brushes and five were sonic. The sonic devices typically come with chargers while the rotating brushes take 2-4 AA batteries.

1. <u>Clarisonic (sonic) - 5.0 Stars / $100-$260</u>

Clarisonic is well known as has a loyal following. Much like Botox, every competitor wants to say they are 'as good as Clarisonic.' That should tell you something right away. This was the best of all exfoliating devices I reviewed. While Clarisonic knows people are willing to pay for quality, they do offer less expensive options. Those who have purchased this product are quick to say it pays for itself. It comes with a 1-3 year warranty depending on the device you buy. Some with sensitive skin may find this brush head to be a bit abrasive when used too frequently. Otherwise, the quality of the product, reliability and ease of use are stellar. This is a high-end device so there are counterfeits out there. I recommend buying from their website or certified retailer.

<u>The Clarisonic Smart Profile</u> comes with heads for both the face and body and has four speeds. It will set you back $265, but comes with a three year warranty. This is what I consider to be the best of the best.

<u>The Clarisonic Mia</u> comes in versions 1, 2 and 3 and they also offer a Mia Fit which is a compact version of the Mia 2.

The Mia 1 ($100) – one speed / 1 year warranty
Mia 2 and Fit ($150) – two speeds / 2 year warranty
Mia 3 ($200) – three speeds / 3 year warranty

Those that use this product rarely complain that it was a waste of money. Here you clearly get what you pay for. Clarisonic (and everyone else) likes to describe their products as working 5-10+ times better than washing your face with your fingertips. I have yet to find a study that supports this claim from Clarisonic or other devices. However, I would agree the Clarisonic does exfoliate more thoroughly than your fingertips. It comes with a rechargeable battery so you don't need to worry about buying batteries.

2. Foreo Luna 2 (sonic) - 4.5 Stars / $200

The silicone head of this brush has a facial cleansing and an anti-aging mode. I really like the unique design here which does allow one to get into tight areas. There are four separate versions, each with a unique design suited for normal, dry, oily or sensitive skin. No need for replacement brushes or batteries. This waterproof unit is very cool indeed and is an up-tick from the standard brush technology. It comes with a 2 year warranty. Like Clarisonic, buy this one from the website or authorized retailer as there are plenty of counterfeits.

3. Beaute La Royale Waterproof Facial Brush (rotating) - 4.0 Stars / $30

Just because a product is inexpensive doesn't *necessarily* mean it is of poor quality. Beaute La Royale's waterproof facial brush comes with four different attachments including a body brush. Users felt as though this was a very good product for so little money and the customer service was the best of any company/product reviewed. It has a true *unlimited warranty.* One user found the unit was not waterproof and received a replacement free of charge. Good customer service goes a long way. Like most of the less expensive products, one minor drawback with the Beaute La Royale is that it comes with only one speed.

4. Silk'n Sonic Clean Plus (sonic) - 4.0 Stars / $90

This system comes with two speed settings, 3 brushes, auto-timer and also offers 'vibrate' and 'pulsate' modes. It is water resistant and is rechargeable, however does not come with a travel case as many other models do. Understand with this model you are paying three times what you may pay for Olay ProX or Beaute La Royale but you do get more as well. Many compare this to the more expensive Clarisonic Mia 2 which *in theory* is a fair comparison. However, when you hold each in your hand you can tell the Clarisonic is a superior device. The Silk'n Sonic comes with a one year warranty.

5. Olay ProX Advanced Cleaning System (rotating) – 4.0 Stars / $35

This is likely one of the best products you will get for about $30. I have used this for many years and can tell you that it is effective and not too abrasive. It also has more than one speed. There is nothing fancy here but perhaps that is what is good about it. Olay ProX is simple and straightforward. This is not a Clarisonic but it is good value for the money. However, its 60 day warranty is far less impressive than some of the other warranties out there. Nonetheless, the ProX I have is over three years old and is doing just fine.

6. Essential Skin Solutions Perfect Skin (rotating) - 3.5 Stars / $30

This is a unit that can be used in the shower or bath and takes 4 AA batteries. Like other models reviewed this has a body brush and pumice head for callouses. This device comes with a cleaning unit, one big body brush, one sensitive skin face brush, a smaller face brush and pumice. The biggest complaint here (similar to other less expensive brushes) was the presence of only one speed. The power with this device tends to be sluggish. There are better and worse. The Essential Skin Solutions is average in many ways, but it is not a bad option for those on a tight budget. Manufacturer says unconditional money back guarantee.

7. Conair True Glow Sonic - 3.5 Stars / $50

This Conair device includes 2 body brushes, 2 facial brushes, a standing charger base and adapter. It feels like a solid unit and comes in three speeds similar to the Clarisonic Mia 3. It is smaller and lightweight and 1/3 the cost of the Mia 2. The brush here is a bit kinder and gentler than the Clarisonic brush as well. One issue with the Conair was an inability to fully charge after several months. My experience is that Conair makes some good products but there is a recurrent problem with durability. It comes with a 1 year warranty. If this brush was more durable it would have been rated much higher. When it is functioning properly it does a fantastic job. However, I would pick many others before the Conair.

8. Clinique Sonic System Purifying Cleansing Brush (sonic) - 3.0 Stars / $95

This sonic cleansing brush is rechargeable and waterproof with two bristle types on the head which is an excellent feature. This has a very lightweight design. Like many less-than-well-made products, this one appears to start out like a real champ then over the course of 3-6 months begins to stop holding a charge or stop working altogether. I would agree with a common complaint that the handle of the brush seems to vibrate more than the brush head. I wouldn't say this was a 'bad' product but you can do much better for around $100. The Clinique sonic comes with a 2 year warranty.

9. Pixnor P2016 (rotating) - 3.0 Stars / $15

This product comes with seven separate heads, three of which are basically soft sponges and one (pumice) which the company claims to be helpful in removing callouses. This seems to be offering quite a bit of bang for a $15 price tag. However, I did give Pixnor three stars since it really was of satisfactory quality. Let's face it (no pun intended) everyone doesn't have the extra cash for a more expensive device. Perhaps this would make a good 'beginner' brush. It comes with a 45 day warranty.

10. The Proactiv Deep Cleansing Brush $65 (rotating) - 1.0 Star / $65

The only reason this brush sells, I presume, is due to the name "Proactive." The makers apparently designed this brush to be used with their products. The internet is littered with complaints (verified reviews) in regard the product not being waterproof, lacking power, breaking down and being cheaply made. This is not worth your time or your $65. Warranty is 60 days. Beaute La Royale had the best customer service and Proactive had the worst.

My Take:

There are quite a few exfoliating devices out there. Physical exfoliation really gives you a great deal of options to consider. I like the sonic devices more than their rotating counterparts. They tend to be solidly made, reliable and far more durable. However, some really like the feeling of the rotating brush. In this case choose Beaute La Royale or Olay ProX. Exfoliation is an important part of any skin care and anti-aging plan and needs to be part of your regimen if you are serious about looking younger. I have no allegiance to any of the products but based on my independent review, I would choose the Clarisonic Smart Profile or Foreo Luna 2.

Microdermabrasion

Microdermabrasion is a modality to remove dead skin cells while stimulating the growth of new vibrant cells. Microdermabrasion is another means to achieve an effective <u>physical exfoliation</u>. This is nothing new by any means. There are many skin resurfacing techniques which have been around for centuries.

- Ancient Egypt – Sour milk (lactic acid) was used as part of a skin rejuvenation regimen (typically only for the wealthy).
- Middle Ages – Old wine (tartaric acid) was used for skin rejuvenation.
- Italy 1985 – Microdermabrasion was first performed.

Microdermabrasion gives results with low risks and literally no downtime. In 2014 it was the #5 medical aesthetic procedure with 417,000 performed.

Microdermabrasion has a huge advantage over chemical peels and laser skin resurfacing in terms of down time and potential side effects. This is because it doesn't penetrate beneath the epidermis. It is important to note that medium to deep chemical peels and laser skin resurfacing **will** penetrate through epidermis into the dermis. In doing so, they clearly confer a more powerful anti-aging benefit. However, a simple microdermabrasion packs a little anti-aging punch of its own.

The Epidermis and Dermis:

- Epidermis: Contains no blood vessels, five layers and no collagen.
- Dermis: Contains blood vessels, supplies the epidermis with nutrients and 70% of the weight of the dermis is due to collagen. Remember, the health of your skin relies heavily on the blood supply to the dermis and what is delivered through it.

The stratum corneum is the outermost layer of the epidermis. It is composed of 15 to 20 thin layers of dead skin cells. These are known as keratinocytes. These old dead cells are continually sloughed off and are replaced by newer cells. As I mentioned, this process slows down from a rate of complete cell turnover of 25-30 days in young adults to 45-55 days in older adults. When there is an excess of dead skin cells, the skin shows more fine lines, wrinkles and a less vibrant complexion.

The reason microdermabrasion has become so accepted and used is because of certain well-known facts:

1. It is quick and painless.
2. There is no downtime or need for anesthesia.
3. It can be used on all skin types.

Understanding the Procedure

- Your face should be cleansed thoroughly.
- The hand held microdermabrasion device begins to function as it touches your skin.
- Crystals (aluminum oxide) are pushed at a high pressure through a tube into the upper layer of skin.
- As the skin cells are removed, so too are the crystals through a vacuum device connected to the machine.

Newer Devices:

Aluminum oxide crystal microdermabrasion systems

These systems have been around for over 20 years. Aluminum oxide is the second hardest mineral, second only to diamonds.

Diamond tip microdermabrasion

These systems replace the aluminum oxide crystals with a diamond tip wand. This offers the advantage of allowing closer approximation to the eyes, mouth and nose. These systems also reduce the risk of stray crystals entering and irritating these areas. Otherwise, in many ways, diamond tip microdermabrasion machines are very similar to aluminum oxide crystal machines. They come with wands of variable size and coarseness for different depths of resurfacing. The wand tip is made of natural laser cut diamond chips which polish the skin, remove dead cells and are vacuumed up.

What Microdermabrasion Helps:

1. Fine lines or wrinkles
2. Age spots, uneven pigmentation or other sun damage
3. Minor scars or uneven skin texture
4. Acne and acne scars – Acne is caused largely by pores blocked with dead skin cells. Microdermabrasion can help to clear clogged pores of dead cells, oil and dirt. I do not recommend microdermabrasion when acne is extremely inflamed. Think of microdermabrasion as a tool to be used to aid in the treatment of acne and minor acne scars. More aggressive skin treatments including chemical peels and laser skin resurfacing are needed to treat deeper acne scars. Acne needs to follow a full skin care and dietary regimen for the best results.
5. Rosacea – The skin with rosacea is characterized by redness, swelling and pimples. I prefer other means for the treatment of rosacea (discussed in chapter 9). However, microdermabrasion has been shown to be helpful as part of the treatment for rosacea in many cases.

Poor Candidates and Precautions:

In the big picture, microdermabrasion is a very safe procedure. However, there are certain situations where it should not be performed. These include severe rosacea, inflamed (active) acne, dermatitis, keloids or those prone to keloid formation or when herpes simplex infection is present. Those with auto-immune diseases or diabetes should speak with their doctor before undergoing microdermabrasion and it should not be performed when pregnant. If you have had facial waxing, artificial tanning, Botox or dermal fillers you should wait 2- 3 weeks before you undergo microdermabrasion. On the other hand, having a microdermabrasion *before* receiving a Botox or dermal filler treatment is a great idea.

The procedure itself is very painless. Sometimes it may feel a little warm as the crystals are peeling away the dead skin cells. The new skin cell layer exposed after microdermabrasion may, for the novice, feel a bit sensitive and warm. Application of a hyaluronic acid containing moisturizer post-procedure is helpful to calm and hydrate the skin.

Cost and Frequency of Treatments

Each treatment takes from 30-60 minutes (hence the name 'lunch hour facial') and costs between $75-200 with an average cost of approximately $150. For the best results multiple treatments are recommended (6-12) spaced apart by 2-4 weeks.

Do it yourself?

Microdermabrasion machines, whether they be diamond tip or aluminum oxide crystals are performed by doctors but more commonly by nurses and aestheticians. These are experts in the field who (hopefully) have been well trained on the use of this machine that gives a medical grade physical exfoliation of the skin.

Many people love the personal care and pampering that comes with a microdermabrasion and facial. Others find it to be expensive and inconvenient. Many have chosen to perform home-based versions. While microdermabrasion was the 5th most popular medical aesthetic treatment in 2014, it was also the only treatment to show a decline in the industry in the past five years. My preference is for people to have a microdermabrasion with a skin care professional, however, the reality is there are plenty of home microdermabrasion machines out there. Hence, the topic warrants some discussion.

Home microdermabrasion systems.

The primary difference between at home vs. professional systems is related to the suction power and whether they are 'diamond tip' or 'aluminum oxide microcrystal' systems. True, diamond tip systems are the *new and improved* version of the aluminum microcrystal systems which have been used for decades. The dermabrasion tips of these machines are etched with tiny diamond chips and offer a very effective means of exfoliation.

Diamond tip microdermabrasion machines are now available for home use. Ideally they will rejuvenate, smoothen and refine the skin. The diamond tip wand with these systems allows for the ability to get closer to the eyes, nose and mouth. Diamond tip systems can give a non-surgical skin exfoliation to peel away the dead skin cells, while vacuum/suction removes dirt, oil and dead skin cells.

The primary reason to purchase an at-home diamond tip microdermabrasion device is cost savings and convenience. Many, (but not all) of these products come with a DVD which is important to watch to fully understand the product you will be using. However, they all come with very clear instruction manuals. Those with severe acne, rosacea, eczema or any other skin infection should speak to their doctor before using these devices. Used properly they can be an effective anti-aging tool. If one is careless, severe skin irritation, scarring or infection can result. I include the review of these products to give you some insight and what to look for if indeed you are considering this option.

1. The New Spa Portable Diamond Microdermabrasion Kit (4.5 stars)

This device does a good job of improving skin tone, smoothness and pore size. Despite its higher rating, the New Spa did not cost more than any other diamond tip microdermabrasion device. This was overall the best device for home microdermabrasion in terms of ease of use, results, suction power and continued reliability. A good friend of mine who battles chronic adult acne found this product helpful in controlling her acne and continued improvement of acne scarring.

2. Kendal Professional Diamond Microdermabrasion System (4.0 stars)

Most of those with experience using this Kendal device found its performance to be very good while being simple and easy to use. One aesthetician I spoke with gave her clients the option of a reduced cost ($65) when she used this device instead of her professional microdermabrasion system. In this situation, people were pleased with the results and the lower cost. In regard to at-home machines, those who had problems with the Kendal found customer service to be very helpful.

3. PMD Personal Microdermabrasion System (non-diamond tip device) (4.0 stars)

PMD makes professional diamond tip microdermabrasion systems for office use for about $1500. This review is for their hand held home microdermabrasion device which runs about $200. This is a quality device which works very well however did lose suction power after 6 months of use on several occasions. I liked the fact that this device came with an excellent DVD training disc.

4. The Nubrilliance Microdermabrasion Skin Care System (3.0 stars)

This was the least impressive. There were issues with broken parts arriving and a noticeable reduction in suction following 3-5 uses. Customer service was felt by many to be sub-par.

Cost – The home treatments mentioned above are all about $200. It really depends on where you are purchasing the device. I would shy away from buying used machines on EBay and the like. If you understand the machine you are using very well and use it properly, it will pay for itself in 2-3 treatments.

Power – The suction power needed for an effective microdermabrasion with these home devices is 16Hg. New Spa has a professional-grade machine with suction up to 25Hg, but really 16Hg is plenty of suction to accomplish a beautiful exfoliation.

Verdict – Understand how to use the microdermabrasion device you choose. Regular home treatments will give you a beautiful exfoliation which ultimately will lead to removal of dead skin, clearance of pores and reduction in pore sizes and fine lines. The removal of the top skin surface with the exfoliation that occurs gives you a boost of new fresh cell growth. This procedure is helpful in bringing a clear and vibrant complexion. My opinion is that home-based treatments for microdermabrasion come with an increased risk of complications. Aestheticians, as a general rule, are experts in the art of exfoliation. Seeing an aesthetician for a microdermabrasion is my preference. However, if cost is an issue and you do your homework on the device you are using, home-based microdermabrasion is a viable option for many.

Chemical Exfoliation

With chemical exfoliation the chemical (acid) is doing the exfoliating work. Amongst the go-to chemical exfoliation agents are the alpha and beta hyroxy acids. These are friends to our chemical exfoliation plan. Glycolic acid is the most commonly used alpha hydroxy acid. The reason behind its widespread use is its small molecular size. This allows for deeper penetration into the skin. When a chemical agent is able to penetrate deeply, it effectively clears unwanted dead skin cells. Salicylic acid is the most commonly used beta hydroxy acid and works particularly well for acne prone skin. Many of the products available contain combinations of physical exfoliants (i.e. microbeads) with salicylic acid. Here you are combining physical and chemical exfoliation factors. The chemical exfoliant acids work by helping to remove the 'glue' that is binding the dead skin cells to the pores and healthy skin cells beneath.

Most experts agree that chemical exfoliation should be no more than two to three times a week and less often if you have sensitive skin. If you are visiting your aesthetician for a stronger chemical exfoliation (a chemical peel) this should be limited to once or twice a month. Again, exfoliating more often or more aggressively with hard scrubbing is not going to help in the big picture.

Chemical Peels

Exfoliation removes dead skin cells thereby allowing lighter, brighter and more vibrant skin to grow. Chemical peels do a fabulous job of exfoliation … and so much more. Remember, exfoliation can be physical; using a product with beads, microbeads or powder to clear away dead skin cells (commonly with the aid of a rotating or sonic pad), or chemical, where the chemical itself does the work.

Chemical peels are divided into three broad categories; superficial (light), medium and deep. In addition to beautiful exfoliation, deeper peels are able to clear unwanted pigment, improve acne (including acne scarring) and remove fine lines and wrinkles. They penetrate the skin; through the epidermis (top layer) to the dermis (layer beneath epidermis) and beyond. Deeper chemical peels can stimulate fibroblasts which improve the structure (collagen) and elasticity (elastin) of the skin.

Have a Realistic Goal

A chemical peel can bring many benefits to your skin. However, they will not reduce the appearance of blood vessels and typically results are not immediate. Peels have to be tailored to the individual and his/her skin type and medical history. The results come as your skin rejuvenates and heals. Though you will get results, many times repeated peels are necessary. Also, deeper, more aggressive peels come with a much longer downtime.

The factors that determine the type and strength of the chemical peel are:

1. The chemical used
2. The percentage (strength) of the chemical
3. How long it is applied
4. The PH level attained (how acidic the peel is). A more acidic peel has a lower PH and will typically result in a deeper

chemical peel. If the PH is less than 2.5, the peel should be performed by a doctor, nurse or aesthetician. Peels with a higher PH can be done in day spas, beauty salons or at home. Remember, as the PH decreases there is an *exponential* increase in peel strength. A peel with a PH of 1.0 is ten times more powerful than one with a PH of 2.0.

Superficial/Light Chemical Peels

Don't be fooled into the belief that a superficial peel need not be taken seriously. With any chemical peel you are putting acid on the skin. This carries with it the potential for side effects. Peels cannot be used on everyone. Superficial peels remove the top layer (epidermis) and it is here where your dead skin cells reside.

Commonly used ingredients are alpha hydroxyl acids (AHAs) like glycolic, lactic or citric acid and beta-hydroxy-acids (BHAs) like salicylic acid. Fruit enzymes from papaya, pineapple, pumpkin and cranberry can be used for light chemical peels as well. Tartaric acid (from grapes) and malic acid (from apples and pears) are milder than glycolic. They remove dead cells, increase cell renewal while clearing oil (sebum).

Advantages of superficial peels:

1. There is minimal down time, other than skin redness (erythema), which typically only lasts a few days.
2. They are essentially painless except for some very mild tingling and burning which may occur.
3. They are the safest and problems such as scarring, infection or pigment changes are rare.

Disadvantage: Multiple treatments are typically needed (6-10) to achieve desired results.

Superficial peels will help to reduce fine lines and wrinkles, fade mild hyperpigmentation and improve acne scarring.

Medium Depth Chemical Peels

Medium depth peels penetrate further, removing much of the epidermis as well as some of the dermis. These peels are more painful and have a much longer down time than superficial peels. The skin may remain red for several weeks or longer until the skin is fully healed. In many cases a light peel will be used prior a medium peel. This helps the medium peel to penetrate more deeply into the dermis. Commonly used ingredients include Trichloroacetic Acid (TCA), Jessner peel (combination of resorcinol, salicylic acid and glycolic acid) or higher concentrations of glycolic acid (50%).

Advantages: More dramatic results in fewer treatments.

Disadvantages: There is more burning and stinging of the face. It may remain swollen, pink, and irritated with more 'peeling' of skin for weeks or longer. As the pigment is cleared you may get brown patches on your skin.

Medium peels help clear melasma or other unwanted pigment. They work well to reduce fine lines and wrinkles. A Jessner peel does exceptionally well in treating both acne and acne scarring.

Deep Chemical Peels

Deep peels do just that, they go deep; through the epidermis and dermis down to the subcutaneous (deepest) skin layer.

Ingredients in deep peels include phenol (carbolic acid) or high concentrations of trichoroacetic Acid (TCA). These acids penetrate deeply through the skin layers.

Advantages: excellent clearing of sun damage, scarring, fine lines and deep wrinkles with the fewest needed treatments.

Disadvantages include pain and a month or longer for full recovery. Excessive redness, swelling, scabbing, itching and peeling are commonly present. Deep peels have the highest incidence of post-procedure pigment issues and scarring.

Deep peels improve fine lines as well as deep wrinkles, scars, sun damage and pre-cancerous growths. I am not prone to recommend deep chemical peels. With the many laser options available, there are other effective ways to reduce fine lines and wrinkles and sun damage without the pain and downtime associated with deep chemical peels. This is just my preference, but as we will discuss in chapter 8, there are laser procedures such as intense pulsed light (IPL) which do a fantastic job of clearing unwanted pigment with very little downtime.

Relative Strengths:

It is important to understand that the peel strength (percentage) does not equate to how deep the peel will penetrate through the skin layers. For instance, 30% glycolic acid is a light peel whereas 30% trichloroacetic acid (TCA) is a deep peel.

- A TCA of 10% and Glycolic of 30% are light peels
- A TCA of 20% and Glycolic of 50% are medium peels
- A TCA of 30% and Glycolic of 70% are deep peels
- A Jessner Peel is considered a medium strength peel.

Skin Types and Safety:

Skin types are defined by what is well known in dermatology circles as the Fitzpatrick scale:

The Fitzpatrick Scale		
Fitzpatrick	Characteristics	Skin type
Type I	Never tans, always burns	Extremely fair skin
Type II	Occasionally tans, usually burns	Fair skin
Type III	Tans average, sometimes burns	Medium skin
Type IV	Usually tans, rarely burns	Olive skin
Type V	Mostly tans, almost never burns	Dark brown skin
Type VI	Never burns	Black skin

The best candidates for chemical peels are the light skin types (I, II and III). These carry less chance for complications such as hyperpigmentation (dark spots), hypopigmentation (light spots) and scarring. Although skin types V and VI are not ideal for chemical peels, they may undergo peels through the use of superficial agents such as salicylic acid or a low percentage glycolic acid (30%).

People with history of scarring (keloids), recent facial surgery, prior sensitivities to peels, auto-immune disorders, aspirin allergy, herpes, or are pregnant or nursing should not have chemical peels. A good doctor, nurse or aesthetician should do a thorough medical history before giving you a chemical peel of *any* strength.

Having even a mild peel will make your skin much more prone to burn. Please be sure to apply your SPF of 50 vs. UVA and UVB rays the days and weeks following your peel. Regardless of your desired goal with a skin peel, leaving your skin unprotected after a peel will not only make it burn more easily, it will provide the perfect skin environment for development of sun spots.

Chemical peels can give amazing results. They are able to effectively exfoliate the skin through removal of dead skin cells, clearance of pores and stimulation of collagen resulting in a lighter, brighter, tighter and more vibrant complexion. We have discussed many means of both physical and chemical exfoliation. These work very well indeed. There are also laser procedures which can be used to bring about exfoliation as well. In chapter 8 we will discuss the many lasers that are available and discuss how they can be used to bring amazing anti-aging results. They can exfoliate, clear red and brown discolorations, shrink pore size, stimulate collagen, reduce the appearance of scars and smoothen out fine lines and wrinkles.

The VI Peel

The VI Peel (Vee-eye-peel) is a chemical peel shown to be effective in the treatment of several troublesome skin issues such as acne, acne scarring, fine lines, wrinkles, enlarged pores, uneven skin pigment and age spots. The fact that the VI Peel penetrates into the dermis means that it also stimulates collagen production to improve skin firmness. The VI Peel brings the benefits of traditional chemical peels but its unique combination of ingredients offers marked results with less downtime. For these reasons the VI Peel is a favorite of both aestheticians and patients.

What exactly is a VI Peel?

A VI peel is made up of a unique mixture of acids, vitamins and other ingredients. Specifically trichloroacetic acid (TCA) 7%, salicylic acid 2%, retinoic acid (vitamin A) 8%, glycolic acid, phenol and vitamin C. Retinoic acid (vitamin A), is well known for its anti-aging, antioxidant and anti-wrinkle attributes. In addition, the presence of vitamin A and salicylic acid are incredibly helpful to those with acne-prone skin. Vitamin C is an antioxidant which stimulates collagen and is well known for its ability to fade unwanted pigment. A VI peel really brings the power of a moderate chemical peel with far less downtime.

What to Expect When You Get a VI Peel:

There is very little preparation needed prior to receiving a VI peel. However, you should avoid UV ray exposure ideally for a week before a VI peel. Your face will be cleansed to remove all traces of oil and dirt. The peel is applied in two separate layers which help to penetrate both the epidermis and dermis. There is very little discomfort with the application of this peel other than some mild stinging or burning. The procedure itself typically takes less than 30 minutes. The peel must remain on your skin for four hours to allow for the peel to fully absorb into the skin layers. During this time you can resume normal activities. After four hours it is recommended that the peel be washed off using a gentle cleanser.

What to Expect After the VI Peel:

- In the first 24-48 hours, despite the peel having been cleansed from the surface of your skin, the chemicals continue to work on your epidermis and dermis.
- At about 72 hours your skin will begin to peel and this will continue for the next 1-3 days.
- By day 5-6 peeling will fully subside. As part of the post-VI peel kit, you will receive the VI Derm moisturizer which can be used to help your skin with the post-peel healing process.
- You need to avoid your typical exfoliating routine until the peeling has subsided. The VI peel is doing aggressive exfoliation for you already.
- Any chemical peel will make your skin more susceptible to damaging UVA/UVB rays, so the use of sunblock SPF 50 is recommended.

People have seen VI peels available online and have asked me if this peel is OK for home use. My strong recommendation is that this and any other chemical peel should be administered only by an experienced skin care professional. VI Peels can be performed every two-three weeks until desired results are achieved.

VI Peel Benefits:

- Reduction of fine lines and wrinkles
- Reduction in unwanted pigment including age spots, uneven pigment and melasma
- Improvement of acne and acne scarring
- Improved texture and tone. Remember the VI peel is able to penetrate into the dermis which allows for improved collagen formation.
- Improved skin clarity and vibrancy.

The VI peel is an excellent option to consider if you are looking for the benefits of a medium chemical peel with less downtime. While it has been stated that this peel may be used on any skin type, I would recommend particular caution on darker skin types (Fitzpatrick V, VI).

Chapter Five

Diet and Wellness

I have made much reference in previous chapters regarding the importance of diet and its role in anti-aging. The right diet is essential to achieving your goal of a youthful, vibrant and beautiful appearance. Any anti-aging plan is incomplete without it. Diet is about treating the skin from the inside-out.

However, much attention is given to treating the skin from the outside-in. There are amazing results to be achieved through cosmetic procedures and the use of the right skin care ingredients. The options available increase every year. The epidermis and dermis of our skin are the targets of the vast majority of these treatments. In the following chapters much attention will be given to the amazing results that Botox, dermal fillers and cosmetic laser treatments can bring to your overall appearance. The results are simply amazing. Skin care applied topically to our skin containing the right ingredients and antioxidants are of utmost importance to the maintenance of a youthful appearance. These outside-in treatments are VERY important. However, those with the very best skin work to treat their skin from the inside-out as well.

The good news is treatment from the inside-out is quite universal and frankly much more straightforward. The right dietary ingredients will help nearly any skin condition. Oxygen, nutrients, and antioxidants are vitally important to the health and wellness of the dermis and epidermis. These are delivered via capillaries in the dermis. By choosing the right ingredients in your diet, most skin conditions improve along with noticeable anti-aging results. The phrase 'you are what you eat' is so very true when it comes to our skin.

In my mind, the days of the traditional food pyramids of the 70s and 80s are over. These are being summarily replaced by modern ideas about what is *truly* a healthy diet for your body and for your skin. The Clear Skin diet is certainly a new pyramid and is likely quite different from what you may have seen growing up. The old pyramid essentially supported large amounts of carbohydrates, a moderate amount of vegetables and lesser amounts of protein. In fact, this is really not what is best for your body and your skin.

A growing number of friends, family, clients, colleagues and ClearSkinMD.net followers are seeing marked skin (and wellness) improvements through following this plan. Think about it. If your diet helps your *skin look better*, don't you think it's making *the rest of your body* better as well? You have heard 'the eyes are the window to the soul?' It is my opinion that the skin is the window to the body.

Healthy Diet = Healthy Body = Healthy Skin

The Clear Skin Diet

I divide dietary factors that will help your skin into five important groups. Before discussing these groups we need to discuss … water.

Water

Understandably water is not a 'food group' but it is discussed first for a very good reason. Water is as important as any other group. Every day you lose water through perspiration, respiration and the urinary / intestinal tract. Your body is (on average) 60% water so it (and your skin) requires a steady supply. Hydrated skin is happy skin. Sufficient water is a vital part of your diet. So how much water does your body need? The Institute of Medicine and Food and Nutrition Board suggest roughly 2 liters per day for women and 3 liters for men. This doesn't take into account weight or activity. I prefer to make it simple. 2 liters is about 68 ounces. Four 16 ounce glasses of water is 64 ounces so my recommendation is **four to five 16 ounce glasses of water each day.**

When you incorporate the fruits and vegetables of this diet you will gain water there as well. For example, cantaloupe, strawberries, pineapple, apples, oranges, lettuce, cabbage, celery and spinach are over 80% water. Granted, this is not the 'same' as water. However, it is important to realize that many healthy foods are also very hydrating to your body and your skin.

When you are dehydrated, your skin suffers. It is dry, secretions are thicker and pores are more easily blocked. The fact of the matter is most people by and large do not drink enough water, nor do they get enough fruits and vegetables. So the first part of the Clear Skin Diet calls for four to five 16 ounce glasses a day. Put some lemon in that water for some antioxidant vitamin C power as well. The water and vitamin C help to flush out toxins from your body. I encourage people to drink one of these glasses of water before each meal. Without a doubt, drinking a glass of water before a meal makes you far less hungry.

What is a Serving?

In terms of fruits and vegetables, it is best understood by considering one serving of fruits and vegetables as 1 cup or approximately the size of your fist. If the fruits or vegetables are chopped, one serving is closer to a half cup.

Polyphenols –You've seen them

Did you ever notice that some fruits and vegetables just catch your eye? The bright colors of fruits and vegetables such as broccoli, spinach, strawberries, raspberries and blueberries are nature's way of signaling to you that these are packed with antioxidant-rich polyphenols. Groups 1 (green leafy vegetables) and group 2 (vitamin A and C-rich fruits) have plenty of these polyphenols.

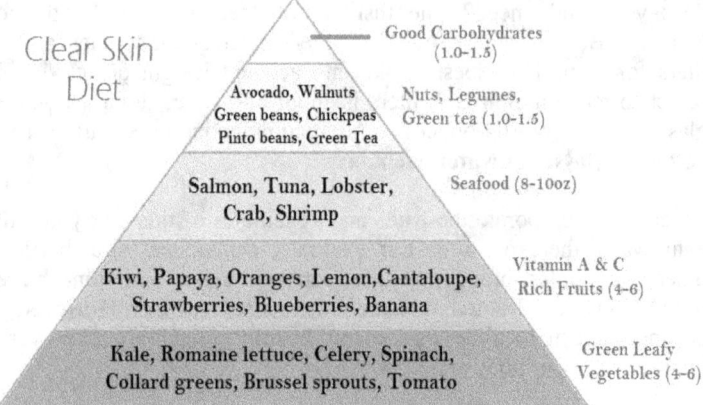

Clear Skin Diet

Good Carbohydrates (1.0-1.5)

Avocado, Walnuts, Green beans, Chickpeas, Pinto beans, Green Tea — Nuts, Legumes, Green tea (1.0-1.5)

Salmon, Tuna, Lobster, Crab, Shrimp — Seafood (8-10oz)

Kiwi, Papaya, Oranges, Lemon, Cantaloupe, Strawberries, Blueberries, Banana — Vitamin A & C Rich Fruits (4-6)

Kale, Romaine lettuce, Celery, Spinach, Collard greens, Brussel sprouts, Tomato — Green Leafy Vegetables (4-6)

<u>Group 1 – Green Leafy Vegetables</u> (4-6 servings)

(Arugula, kale, collard greens, Brussel sprouts, chard, romaine lettuce, celery and spinach)

Why they is necessary in your diet:

- Lots of vitamin A – a fabulous anti-oxidant
- Chlorophyll - clears bacteria and toxins from the digestive tract
- Zeaxanthin – (in cooked spinach) brings strong anti-oxidant properties.
- This food group is loaded with antioxidants and foods that stabilize hormone levels.

Why this helps:

- Anything in your diet with vitamin A is going to be helpful to combat acne and regenerate skin. Other foods with vitamin A include carrots, papaya, tomatoes, watermelon and apricots.
- Free radicals form in your skin in response to a multitude of environmental factors ultimately destroying the cell membrane and altering the cell DNA. Antioxidants neutralize free radicals and stimulate collagen production, repair cells and have anti-inflammatory properties to fade redness.

- Fluctuations in certain hormones have been shown to trigger acne breakouts and slow the natural regenerative processes of your skin. Green leafy vegetables help to stabilize these hormones.

Group 2 – Vitamin A and C-rich Fruits (4-6 servings)
(Oranges, Kiwi, Papaya, Lemon, Cantaloupe, Strawberries, Blueberries, Bananas)

What they have: vitamin A, vitamin C and antioxidants

Anti-oxidants in your diet, as mentioned, rid your skin of free radical damage. Vitamin A is a natural anti-acne vitamin and helps regenerate new skin. Vitamin C also fights free radicals, increases collagen, fades unwanted pigment and reduces wrinkles.

Group 3 – Seafood (8-10 ounces, uncooked/before cooking)
(Salmon, Tuna, Lobster, Crab, Shrimp)

What they have: Omega 3 fatty acids

Also known as the 'good fat', these fatty acids help at the level of the individual cell by improving the health of the cell membrane, giving the skin a healthy glow and improved skin texture. Certain components of seafood may also have anti-bacterial qualities and help protect against UVA/UVB rays. Omega 3 fatty acids are also found in walnuts, canola oil and flax seed.

Group 4 – Green Tea, Legumes (beans) and Nuts (1.0-1.5 cups total of legumes and nuts)
(Walnuts, almonds, green beans, pinto beans, chickpeas)

Green Tea is loaded with anti-oxidants and fights inflammation. Drinking one to two 8-oz cups of green tea is simply good for your skin. In chapter 3 we learned green tea contains the polyphenol *'catechin'* which gives green tea serious antioxidant power. Nuts and legumes are high in vitamin E which is a strong antioxidant and wrinkle fighter. They also contain zinc which boosts the immune system.

Group 5 - Good Carbohydrates (and more antioxidants)

When it comes to beauty from the inside-out, good carbs and antioxidants are just what the doctor ordered.

Good Carbs and the Glycemic Index

The glycemic index (GI) is a way to measure the carbohydrates of different foods and their impact on blood sugar and insulin release. Simply put, foods with a high GI cause a sharp rise in blood sugar. When your body absorbs sugars quickly, the pancreas secretes insulin in response. The problem is that the release of insulin produces inflammatory cells and encourages your body to store fat.

Put another way, when you eat foods high in sugar or those quickly converted to sugar (i.e. bad carbs) this results in an excessive amount of sugar entering the blood stream. Your body really has no other option than to store this excess sugar as fat. This whole process is hard on your body and most certainly your skin.

Fried foods are quite problematic too for different reasons. The processed plant oils used in frying oxidize at high frying temperatures. This oxidation releases free radicals and makes circulation sluggish everywhere, including your skin. Anything you consume that is increasing the load of free radicals and reducing circulation is going to be harmful to your body as well as your skin. It is worth mentioning again, free radicals and poor circulation are two strong contributing factors to aging skin.

Making dietary choices with a lower glycemic index will thereby aid your skin in several ways.

1. The foods themselves do not *add* to the presence of free radicals, they will *neutralize* them.
2. By reducing the rate of insulin release, low glycemic index foods are helping to improve circulation.
3. A diet rich in antioxidants with a low glycemic index results in less inflammation. Since we know inflammation is harmful to your skin, anything to reduce it is skin-friendly.

The chart on the following page is a guide that I have devised which mirrors the current research in anti-aging and skin care. The focus here is to choose foods with a low glycemic index. These are commonly referred to as 'good carbs.' Powerhouse antioxidants prevent rapid insulin release *and* give your skin a strong antioxidant punch from the inside-out. This is not to say that bananas, pineapple and watermelon are 'bad' for you. They tend to be higher in sugar and lower in antioxidant power than many other foods listed.

When choosing carbohydrates of the 'bread/cereal and grain' variety, it is always better to choose 'whole grains.' Stay away from white bread, rice or pasta. The body tends to break these rapidly into sugars. Also steer clear of non-whole-grain waffles, sugary cereals and pancakes.

We all want to look and feel younger. There is a large overlap between the list of good carbs and antioxidant powerhouses. Your body wants polyphenols, a diet rich in antioxidants and foods that do not cause a sharp rise in your insulin levels. It takes consistency and without a doubt, the right diet will help your skin be beautiful from the inside-out.

www.GlycemicIndex.com provides diet and recipes including low carbohydrate (low glycemic index) and high antioxidant foods. It is definitely worth a look.

Good Carbs / Bad Carbs and Powerhouse Antioxidants
Glycemic Index = GI

Foods	Low GI (Good Carbs)	High GI (Bad Carbs)	Powerhouse Antioxidants
Vegetables	Asparagus Bell Peppers Bok Choy Broccoli Brussel Sprouts Cabbage/Kale Cauliflower Celery Collard Greens Cucumbers Tomatoes Turnip Greens Spinach Summer Squash	Beets Carrots Corn Potatoes Sweet Potatoes	Bell Peppers Spinach Summer squash Kale Turnip Greens Brussel Sprouts Cantaloupe Blueberries Strawberries Honeydew Melon
Fruits	Blueberries Strawberries Cantaloupe Honeydew Melon Kiwi Fruit Peaches/Pears Oranges Lemon/Lime	Banana Apricot Fig Papaya Pineapple Raisins Watermelon Fruit "Juices"	
Seafood	Salmon Cod Shrimp Tuna	(Red Meat)	**Omega 3-Rich** Salmon Shrimp Tuna
Poultry/Lamb	Pasteur raised Chicken / Grass fed Lamb		
Eggs/Dairy	Pasture raised eggs/ Yogurt	Whole milk 2% milk	

Food Allergies and Your Diet

Many chronic skin conditions can be attributed to or exacerbated by certain foods. Researchers estimate that nearly 15 million Americans have some type of food allergy. 90% of food allergies are attributed to seven foods: ***dairy, eggs, peanuts, tree nuts, gluten, fish and shellfish.*** In the worst case scenario food allergies can even be life threatening. If you think you are having a food allergy, of course call 911 or go to the emergency room. Many people suspect they are allergic to certain foods and limit or omit them from their diet. In many cases this may not be necessary. I recommend anyone who feels they may have a food allergy consult with a physician. The doctors most capable of identifying food allergies are *allergy and immunology specialists.* An excellent website to visit to better understand food allergies is www.foodallergy.org.

When it comes to diet, I like for people to approach it much like exercise. Don't try to change (or do) everything all at once. If you begin an overly aggressive path it is very difficult to maintain. Be aware of what is helpful to your skin and continue to make positive changes in your diet, while reducing foods known to do nothing but add free radicals for your body to fight.

It takes the average person six weeks to develop a new healthy habit. Many quit because they do not see results right away. When you make a decision to follow this diet, give it a full six weeks. Mark your calendar.

Before starting any new diet you should consult your physician to make certain there are no contraindications to doing so with your current health or medications you may be taking. You can get there, the key is consistency. Any person who looks healthy with beautiful skin did not begin their journey last week. Further, those who are most successful continually ask themselves, "Is this food or lifestyle choice going to help or hurt my skin?"

Superstar Skin Supplements

Every day our skin is exposed to a multitude of environmental insults and free radicals. Through the years this culminates in sun damage, loss of collagen, larger pores, poor skin texture, fine lines, wrinkles and loose skin.

The push for medication through advertisements is more present than it has been ever in the history of medicine. The father of medicine, Sir William Osler noted, "The person who takes medicine must recover twice, once from the disease and once from the medicine." Hence, I am not a fan of prescription medicine unless absolutely necessary. Vitamin supplements are a completely different story. These are *nutrients* which are helpful to your body and your skin.

Skin Supplements that Help Your Skin:

1. Antioxidants

There are many antioxidant skin supplements. These neutralize free radicals, stimulate collagen production, repair cells and fade redness. Our skin makes its own antioxidants and tries desperately to keep up and clear away all the free radicals but commonly falls short of neutralizing them. Similar to how we use antioxidants topically, we can also help our skin with antioxidant skin supplements. Whether these free radical-fighters are in our diet as foods or supplements, they will enter our blood stream and make their way to the dermal capillaries where they exert their anti-aging effect on the dermis and epidermis.

- **Vitamin A** – The benefits of vitamin A are wide and varied. From a physiologic standpoint, it is best known for benefits to the eyes, skin and immune system. In the skin it helps acne, eczema, psoriasis, cold sores, sunburn and helps with healing of wounds and burns. The typical dose is 3000 micrograms (10,000 units) once daily and should be used with caution if you are taking antibiotics or blood thinners. Other excellent dietary sources of vitamin A are sweet potatoes, carrots, dark leafy greens, lettuce, dried apricots, fish, cantaloupe, tropical fruits and bell peppers.

- **Vitamin C** – This is one of my favorite skin supplements. While the best way to help your skin with vitamin C is to put it *on* your skin; vitamin C as a supplement is an excellent antioxidant which helps to improve the absorption of vitamin E and iron. The recommended dose for men is 90 milligrams/day and for women 75 milligrams/day. Fresh vegetables and citrus fruits contain lots of Vitamin C (Clear Skin diet group 3).

- **Vitamin E-** Similar to vitamin C, vitamin E is an antioxidant that neutralizes the free radicals that can cause fine lines and wrinkles. Most people get plenty in their diet and too much vitamin E can cause bruising. Other sources include avocado, olive oil and wheat germ.

- **Acai Berry** – This antioxidant has gained momentum in recent years. It brings strong antioxidant power. It also contains fatty acids such as oleic acid which, like omega 3 fatty acids, helps to nourish and protect the skin.

- **PL Extract** – This is the new kid on the block. The long name for this antioxidant is *polypodium leucotomos* (PL) extract. You will find this product marketed under the trade name *Heliocare*. Experts agree that this offers the equivalent of SPF 8 protection if taken once daily. It is reasonable then to conclude that PL extract will help your sun block work more effectively and help to 'cover' areas you may have missed when applying sun block. A study in the Journal of Clinical and Aesthetic Dermatology in 2014 showed that PL extract, when used for three months, helped fade hyperpigmentation and melasma.

2. Biotin

Biotin, a B-Vitamin, is typically known for how it improves brittle nails and hair. Biotin deficiency can result in dermatitis, eczema and psoriasis.

In theory these same skin conditions are felt to improve through the use of biotin. The recommended dose is 2.5 mg/day. Peanut butter and bananas are excellent sources of biotin.

3. Glucosamine

Glucosamine is a naturally occurring substance that is found in fluid in the body's joints. It is well known for its role in building cartilage and has been used for many years to help the symptoms associated with arthritis.

Glucosamine is also beneficial to our skin. It can be converted into substances called polymers and proteoglycans. These are important components in the formation of glycosaminoglycans (like hyaluronic acid that keeps your skin moist). Proteoglycans can block melanin production and help fade age spots. In 2001, researchers reported that use of an oral supplement containing glucosamine, minerals, and various antioxidant compounds improved the appearance of visible wrinkles and fine lines. The recommended daily dose is 1500mg/day.

Menopause and Your Skin

Menopause, by definition, is when a woman has not had a menstrual period for 12 months. The time leading up to eventual cessation of these periods is referred to as 'perimenopause.' This is marked by the debilitating symptoms of hot flushes, mood swings and sleep disturbances. Women typically go through menopause in their late 40s to early 50s with an average age of 51. Some women pass this phase quite smoothly while others struggle with a troubling myriad of symptoms. Technically 85% of women will experience menopausal symptoms. For most, these symptoms cease within a year but in others may last up to 2-3 years. A decline in estrogen levels is the main contributor to these symptoms, although decreased levels of progesterone and testosterone play an important role as well.

Through perimenopause and menopause the overall trend is for estrogen levels to decrease, however this is not always a *steady* decrease. Women have a wide array of experiences with menopause.

One universal fact is that the reduced amount of estrogen seen with menopause comes with unfavorable changes to the skin.

Menopause and Your skin

1. The Epidermis (top skin layer) becomes thinner and drier.

Estrogens help improve blood flow to the skin through capillaries in the dermis (layer below epidermis). These capillaries supply nutrients and oxygen to the basal layers of the epidermis (where new epidermal cells are being made). With less estrogen, the blood flow to the dermis and epidermis becomes less brisk. This causes a diminished rate of new cell growth. The epidermis then becomes thinner resulting in increased moisture loss and a drier surface. Dry skin means more fine lines and wrinkles.

2. The Dermis has less collagen.

Estrogen plays an important role in protein synthesis. Since collagen is a protein, diminished estrogen levels result in decreased synthesis and repair of the collagen (and elastin) in the dermis. The skin now loses elasticity, tightness and firmness. When the dermal collagen is exposed to environmental insults such as UV rays, the skin struggles to repair the damage. In younger women this repair is much more rapid. With less estrogen, the repair becomes slower resulting in a greater prevalence of fine lines and wrinkles.

3. There is less sub-cutaneous fat.

Estrogens directly affect to how fat is distributed throughout the female body. With a decrease in estrogen comes a decrease of supportive fat below the skin layers of the face and neck. Decreased collagen and supporting fat cells in the tissues beneath it result in fine lines, wrinkles and sagging skin.

4. There are changes in melanin production.

The cells that produce melanin (melanocytes) are *also* regulated by estrogen. With less melanin the skin becomes lighter and more prone to sun damage. Women around the age of menopause (and everyone else) should use sun block with a minimum SPF of 20 on exposed skin, particularly of the face, neck and hands.

5. Acne may rear its ugly head.

During adulthood, with adequate estrogen available, the fluid secreted by sebaceous glands is thin, light and less likely to block pores. At this time, estrogen and testosterone are in balance. During menopause, with a decrease in estrogen the testosterone can exert a greater effect. With more testosterone and less estrogen the sebaceous gland secretions become thick and heavy thereby making the skin more acne prone.

I suspect reading thus far paints a mighty bleak picture … but fear not. There is plenty you can do to help your skin look great despite the diminished estrogen (and progesterone) levels seen during menopause.

Improving Your Skin during Menopause

At its core, medical aesthetics and skin care is about improving the top layer of skin while helping to increase the supporting layers (collagen and elastin). Ideally we achieve a smooth, vibrant epidermal layer with an elastic, toned and firm architecture supporting it. So with menopause we will utilize every possible (and safe) treatment in our arsenal to do just that.

1. Replace the Estrogen

Everyone cannot take estrogen replacement but if you can, this is clearly step #1. This is a hotly contested area especially with the arrival of 'bio-identical hormones' as an alternative. Certain types of cancers including breast or uterine cancer, a history of heart attack/heart disease, stroke, liver disease, or blood clots are conditions which preclude women from taking hormone replacement therapy (HRT). This is something that needs to be approached on an individual basis and discussed at length with your doctor. If no contraindication exists to taking HRT your skin will be much happier with more estrogen around.

2. Avoid Skin Irritants

Changes in humidity, particularly a lower humidity in the winter months can dry out your skin. Wear gloves and a scarf to protect your hands and face from cold and wind in the winter. Keep your thermostat set to 67-70 degrees. Use a humidifier; an optimal humidity level is 45-55%. Keep your showers brief with cooler water and avoid 'scrubbing' your skin. Hot and long showers combined with aggressive scrubbing strips your skin of its protective, moisture preserving oils.

Avoid any soap or shampoo with heavy perfumes which can be irritating to your skin. Unscented is universally better for your skin.

Do not neglect to consider the possibility that bed sheets, clothing, dryer sheets, laundry detergents and shampoos may contain skin irritants. If your skin is newly irritated or dry, try to recall if you have tried a new detergent, shampoo, soap, cleanser or other facial product.

3. Moisturize Your Skin

Hyaluronic acid should be an ingredient somewhere in your daily skin care regimen due to its amazing ability to keep moisture in the skin. It is almost like an anti-wrinkle vitamin. It doesn't end there as the list of effective ingredients to help moisturize and hydrate your skin is lengthy. Some favorites include glycerin, lanolin, ceramides, dimethicone, jojoba oil and coconut oil.

4. Treat Acne if Present

Many women around age 50 may find themselves wandering through the 'acne isle' at the local pharmacy. With a relative increase in testosterone due to the lower levels of estrogen, sebum thickens on what may already be dry skin. This is a recipe for adult acne. While no acne treatment regimen is 'one size fits all' (nothing is like that *anywhere* in medicine for that matter), improvements in diet along with the use of salicylic acid are certain to help. Regular microdermabrasion when the skin is not overly inflamed is another strong consideration. In chapter 9 we discuss effective acne treatments.

5. **Consider procedures known to increase cell turnover and collagen in the skin.**

Three procedures that come to mind are chemical peels, micro needling and laser skin resurfacing. In different ways these treatments all increase new cell production in the epidermis making it thicker and more vibrant while also boosting the amount of collagen in the dermis.

6. **Consider having a medical aesthetic treatment such as Botox or dermal fillers.**

Cosmetic treatments such as Botox or dermal fillers (Restylane, Juvederm or Radiesse) will give you some real and immediate help in reducing fine lines and wrinkles. We discuss Botox and dermal fillers in depth in chapters 6 and 7.

Menopause can be an overwhelming and difficult time in a woman's adult life. I have treated thousands of women around the time of menopause and the changes to the skin are nearly universal. It comes down to a matter of hormone deficiencies affecting nearly every aspect of a woman's life. Weight gain is another issue as are problems with sleep and depression. Amidst these changes the last thing a woman wants to do is look in the mirror and see new fine lines and wrinkles.

By being aware of the causes and following a plan of treatment, there are many ways to keep your skin beautiful through menopause and beyond.

Burning Fat

In chapter 8 we will discuss non-surgical means for fat reduction using lasers. Even with the help of lasers and diet, many people still struggle with excess unwanted fat. The Clear Skin diet focuses on increasing your fruit, vegetable and water intake. Avoidance of foods with a high glycemic index will help to prevent your body's storage of fat. Exercise is an effective means to help clear away unwanted fat as well. In this section we look at ways to beef-up our body's ability to clear away unwanted fat.

1. Drink More Water

I have recommended four to five 16oz glasses of water per day. If you are serious about burning fat, an increased water intake will be helpful. Add another two 16 ounce glasses of water a day for a total of six to seven (or 96-112oz.). Water helps flush toxins from your body. Increased water consumption also reduces hunger.

2. Avoid High Glycemic Index foods

High glycemic index foods such as white rice, breads, sugary cereals, pasta, potatoes and waffles cause a rise in blood sugar and insulin. Some is stored for energy as glycogen but the remainder will be stored as fat. Regardless of your exercise plan, if you are eating too many high glycemic index foods, you are fighting an uphill battle.

3. Avoid Aggressive Calorie Changes

If women cut more than 250 calories from their diet and men cut over 400, the body will sense that it is literally 'starving.' This results in a decrease of the basal metabolic rate (BMR). The BMR reflects the amount of calories you burn throughout a typical day (including sleep). The goal of exercise and fitness is to *increase* the BMR. One of the main reasons 'crash diets' are ineffective is because they *lower* the BMR. Once people return to their regular eating plan, the body lags behind, saving calories since it *perceives* a temporary state of starvation. With a slower BMR, the weight quickly comes back … and then some.

4. Eat More Fruits and Vegetables

Follow the Clear Skin diet and eat 4-6 servings of fruits and 4-6 of vegetables. As noted, many fruits and vegetables have a high percentage of water. They tend to fill you up and help to reduce hunger.

5. Add 25+ mg of Fiber

Increasing fruits and vegetables will certainly add to your daily fiber. Additional fiber absorbs water in your stomach and literally takes up more space which helps to reduce hunger.

6. Exercise and Focus on Fat Burning

Shedding fat requires exercise. For many getting into a regular exercise routine seems like a daunting task. It does not require hard and painful exercise routines; quite the contrary. Exercise does much more than simply burn fat; it increases your basal metabolic rate (BMR). If you are exercising even 30 minutes three times a week, you can improve your BMR. This means that even when you aren't exercising, you are still burning more calories per hour than you were prior.

Fat Burn Zone

There are many complicated calculations available to determine the 'ideal' heart rate needed to burn fat. This simple approach is the way to go. Calculate your fat burn heart rate:

220 – Age = maximal heart rate.
Now multiply this number X (.65) = **Fat burn zone.**
For someone 40 years old:
220 – (**40**) = 180 max heart rate.
Multiply 180 X (.65) = **117.**
So if you are 40 your max heart rate is 180 and your fat burn zone is 117. (+/-4) = **113-121.**

Most machines such as treadmills will offer ways to monitor your heart rate. There are other options available such as wrist heart rate monitors such as Fitbit and Vivofit. This is not an exact science. In the example above, I would recommend trying to stay in the 113-121 range. If the heart rate is a bit above or below that range for a few minutes, adjust your pace.

Most can elevate their heart rate up to a fat burn zone during a brisk (4mph) walk. Do this for 30 minutes three times a week and you are well on your way to burning off your own "pudge" while helping your skin as well. How does exercise help your skin? Ellen Murmur, MD, author and professor of Dermatology at Mt. Sinai School of Medicine states, "By increasing blood flow [to the dermis] exercise helps nourish skin cells and keep them vital. In addition to providing oxygen, blood flow also helps carry away waste products including free radicals."

What I recommend to both friends and clients is to start slow and do something that you are comfortable with to prevent burnout. Then, when you feel up to it, add on more time or more days to your fat burn routine. Exercise has a way of becoming a healthy habit as long as you stay consistent.

Cardio Zone

The cardio zone is much more robust in terms of difficulty and calorie burning potential.

220 – Age = max heart rate.
Now take your max heart rate X **0.8 = Cardio Zone**
Using the 40 year old example:
Multiply (220-40) X 0.8 = 144 (=/- 5)
Cardio zone here would be **139-149.**

Like the name implies, getting into the cardio zone helps your heart. Tasks that used to make you exhausted and short of breath (like climbing a flight of stairs) will become less so, or absent all together as you improve the strength of your heart.

Cardio workouts have also been shown to improve the 'feel good' hormones such as dopamine which improve mood and lessen depression or anxiety. Those who work out and enter fat burning and/or cardio zones show improvements in their metabolism. You burn calories while exercising, but it goes a step further. When you increase your metabolism (BMR) you are actually burning more calories at rest as well.

I have treated many patients who were diabetic due to poor diet and lack of exercise. Through regular (non-painful) exercise, many of them were able to shed pounds and improve their metabolism (BMR). These changes have allowed many to reduce their diabetes medication or discontinue them entirely.

Before starting any exercise routine make sure to check with your doctor. He/she may order and EKG or cardiac stress test to make certain your heart is ready for exercise.

Think Thin and Join a Gym

Getting started on an exercise routine is something that requires a first step. The six week rule applies here as well. Give yourself six weeks to determine if you are able to stick with your routine or need to adjust. Many quit because their workouts are too strenuous or too difficult resulting in burnout. Remember: start now but *slow and steady.*

Sometimes simple changes are a great way to start. Small steps become bigger ones. For instance, at the mall or grocery story, don't look for the closest parking spot. Park your car far away and walk. Take the stairs. Do 30 jumping jacks every morning. Simple changes can reap big rewards long term.

Joining a health club provides some extra motivation for many. Health club memberships have nearly doubled in the past fifteen years. Clubs like LA Fitness, Planet Fitness and Gold's Gym are popular choices for many. Life Time Fitness has taken health clubs to a whole new level. These facilities are really 'healthy way of life destinations.' The presence of indoor and outdoor pools, organic cafes, full service spas *and medical spas* make these locations seem more like wellness destinations (vs. 'the gym'). I foresee these types of wellness centers gaining momentum in the years ahead.

Chapter Six

Botox Cosmetic, Dysport & Xeomin (aka 'The Neurotoxins')

Botox Cosmetic

In 2002 the world of cosmetic medicine changed forever with the introduction of Botox Cosmetic. Botox is a neurotoxin (also referred to as a *neuromodulator*). The toxin itself (*botulinum toxin*) is produced by the bacteria *Clostridium botulinum*. Botox binds reversibly to a nerve. In medical aesthetics this refers to nerves in the face. Nerves innervate muscle. By blocking the nerve, the movement of the muscle is temporarily blocked.

Botox was not originally intended for cosmetic uses. In fact, it came about in quite a round-about way. In the 1990s, it was felt Botox could be useful for neurologic conditions such as bladder spasms, writer's cramp and even cerebral palsy. The most amazing discovery came when a Canadian ophthalmologist, Dr. Jean Carruthers, noticed a reduction in frown lines when using Botox to treat a patient with blepharospasm (an involuntary tight closure of the eyelids).

This was followed by a study in the *Journal of Dermatology and Oncology* in 1992 published by her and dermatologist-husband. The study essentially demonstrated that Botox was a simple and safe procedure for the treatment of brow wrinkles. Many doctors began to use Botox 'off label' for treatment of brow wrinkles, to such a degree that the supply soon ran out.

In 2000, Botox was approved for cervical dystonia (neck/shoulder spasms). In 2002, the FDA approved Botox for use for temporary improvement of glabellar (brow) lines in adult. The last 14 years has seen a steady increase in the use of Botox. It has retained the #1 spot for most sought after and administered medical aesthetic treatment for over a decade.

Why Botox Works

Your face has 43 muscles of variable sizes. When these muscles repeatedly contract tens of thousands of times each year, they literally squeeze the epidermis and collagen-containing dermis until fine lines and wrinkles begin to appear, and deepen. Botox blocks nerve impulses thereby preventing movement of facial muscles in injected areas. In doing so, these fine lines, wrinkles and furrows in the brow, forehead and around the eyes begin to soften. The collagen and elastin fibers can relax, stretch out and smoothen. A common myth is that Botox exerts its effect directly on a wrinkle. The effect on the wrinkle actually comes last. Botox blocks the nerve resulting in diminished facial muscle movement. It is only then that the wrinkle softens or resolves.

Pliability and Elasticity

Skin **pliability** is the ability of the skin to stretch and **elasticity** is the ability of the skin to recoil. Many of the medical aesthetic treatments we use such as chemical peels, microneedling, cosmetic laser treatments (IPL/Fraxel), microdermabrasion and dermal fillers will stimulate fibroblasts to make more collagen and elastin. By doing this we improve the youthful skin features of strength, pliability, and elasticity. The repeated contraction of facial muscles has an adverse effect on the elasticity and pliability of the skin. The main reason for this is largely a loss of collagen and elastin.

In a 2015 study in JAMA Facial Plastic Surgery, Dr. James Bonaparte revealed that the use of Botox made the skin more pliable and elastic. He noted, "We found if we treat people with Botox using standard techniques, we see an increase in elasticity, which is what you'd see in people with more youthful skin ... We're actually seeing evidence that we, for some reason, are getting more elastin and collagen in the skin."

This kind of makes sense. In this study the muscles of the brow and lateral orbital rhytids (crow's feet) were treated. These muscles (when they are moving) are continually pulling on the skin and squeezing the dermis while putting strain on collagen and elastin fibers. Most experts agree with this premise but go a step further. I concur with Dr. Bonaparte's belief that improved pliability and elasticity of the skin may also be related to a receptor in these fibroblasts (or in the collagen itself) that somehow responds to Botox.

The Botox Study Findings Were:

1. Botox increased the stretch and elastic recoil of the women's faces studied. This effect mimicked younger skin.
2. The effect was similar to what was seen with radiofrequency skin tightening, an aesthetic procedure that uses radio waves to heat the dermis causing an increase in collagen and elastin.
3. The tightening and firming features were not a by-product of inflammation or swelling caused by the injections themselves.
4. The effect lasted about four months.

A Difference of Opinion:

Some experts felt the paralysis of the muscles caused by Botox simply gave the collagen and elastin a chance to recover from repetitive muscle movement. Others believe that Botox has an inherent property that stimulates fibroblasts to make collagen and elastin. This is an interesting theory. According to Dr. Bonaparte, "we may be able to develop some medications that don't require injection that you can apply topically and get the same skin rejuvenation effects as Botox." It has become evident that peptides, in particular *neuro*peptides are at the forefront of the discussion of topical ways to achieve results similar to Botox, without the use of a needle. Still other experts feel that repetitive muscle movements create waste products upon which Botox may actually have an antioxidant effect. One study, lots of theories.

My feeling is that Botox's effect on the improved pliability and elasticity of the skin is likely related to the ability of the muscles to 'rest' thereby giving the collagen and elastin a chance to relax and strengthen. Secondly, the actual injection itself may stimulate fibroblasts; similar to what one may see with injection of dermal fillers, micro-needling or radiofrequency skin tightening.

Botox's array of uses extends beyond simple paralysis of facial muscles. It can also cause 'corrective' movements of muscles. If injected in specific locations it can raise the eyebrows or corners of the mouth. It can also treat 'smoker's lines' around the mouth and wrinkles in the chin and neck.

Botox Cosmetic can also be used to reduce excessive sweating (hyperhidrosis) under the arms. In fact, Botox injection to this location results in an 82-87% decrease in sweating. Similar to how Botox blocks the nerves innervating facial muscles, it also blocks the action of sweat glands. Results here may last up to six months or longer.

Getting Botox

Botox has reigned supreme in the medical aesthetic world as the #1 sought after and administered treatment. With beauty so very important and Botox as a means to get there the plan should be simple correct? Just go and get Botox ... Not so fast.

Back in 2005, I had a great deal of experience in primary care medicine and skin care. I had been a doctor for 12 years. If I wanted to, I could order a vial of Botox and inject whomever I wanted, with absolutely no training. The fact that I had an MD after my name was all that was really necessary to administer Botox. I certainly didn't do that. I studied facial muscles more in depth, attended 'hands-on" seminars and then shadowed an experienced plastic surgeon for three months. Only after that time was I ready to administer Botox on real patients. I studied and made drawings of each facial muscle and what each would do if injected.

My point is that many practitioners with little training are injecting. This book is about anti-aging, skin care and looking more youthful. It is also about how to accomplish this goal *safely*. True, finding somewhere to get Botox is not difficult. Finding someone trained well and experienced with neurotoxin injections is another story. The best providers have a deep understanding of facial anatomy, experience and an aesthetic eye for what is the best treatment approach. A red flag should go up when you encounter a new medical spa offering a deep Botox discount. These are a hot-bed for poorly trained injectors out to make a quick buck. Word of mouth is a great avenue to some assurances that the person injecting is qualified. There is also nothing wrong with asking for certifications or licenses. You may feel awkward or timid in doing so. This is a no-brainer. Anyone asking for licensure or explanation of my experience or that of my staff is refreshingly welcome.

Along the same lines, many people are very hesitant to get Botox for fear that their face will become 'frozen.' Celebrities are notorious for having too much Botox and ending up with a 'frozen face.' Many will see these ceramic-faced images in a magazine and swear off Botox for life. In order to achieve the best result both the location and *quantity* of neurotoxin should be administered properly. Over-Botox is not pretty and will last for many months. Make it clear that you want the changes to be subtle. In medical aesthetics, less is more. The object is to enhance your beauty and reverse changes that have come through time. Natural results are the goal – always.

There is no definitive age as to when to come in for a Botox treatment. I have treated women from age 21-70+. Certainly when wrinkles appear, Botox can be helpful. The best results are seen with those who receive Botox every four months. This way, one has a continued smoothening of wrinkles with little or no recurrence. Genetics certainly plays a powerful role in who gets wrinkles where and when. I have no problem treating younger patients as women in their 20s quite commonly have very pronounced brow and forehead wrinkles. Other individuals may be in their mid-40s with very few noticeable wrinkles.

What a Botox Treatment Won't Do for You

For many, the decision to have a cosmetic procedure comes following years of trepidation and worry. People repeatedly weigh the pros and cons before finally 'pulling the trigger' and walking into the medical aesthetic or cosmetic surgeon's office. Many start with Botox or dermal fillers. Why do people come in to have these procedures done in the first place? Most people don't remember the first time they went to a gym or had a haircut, but the first time walking in to a doctor's office for a cosmetic procedure ... *that* they remember.

So tell me ... what brings you in today?

- "I want to look younger."
- "People are telling me I look tired (or angry)."
- "I don't *look* the way I *feel*."
- "I want to do it for myself"

Let's dig a little deeper into these common responses. When people (I am referring to both women *and* men here) want to look younger is there a deeper reason? Or I am making too much ado about nothing?

A study in the Canadian Journal of Plastic Surgery in 2012 showed that certain factors were statistically significant in terms of those willing to have cosmetic procedures. Though more common in women, the results mirrored what is true in the real world. Namely, men are equally as open to having these procedures as women. Men have had a 205% increase in cosmetic procedures in the past five years. Men love Botox as much as women do. Medical aesthetics is gaining incredible momentum across age groups and genders more than ever before.

Specifically, the Canadian journal's study showed those with lower ratings of self-esteem and life satisfaction, were more willing to have cosmetic procedures. Indeed this is a dangerous conclusion. A doctor would certainly never convey that to a patient. "I see you are here for Botox for your low self-esteem!" How dare you! I would say I had my first aesthetic treatment because I felt that my outside was looking a tad older than I felt on the inside. In addition, there is nothing wrong with a little boost in one's self confidence or making subtle changes to help you look your best.

I am the first to say that I love to make people look and feel better. As human beings most all of us have struggled at one point or another with low self-esteem. If you haven't, you are in the minority and consider yourself fortunate. I certainly have, but it is not why I have a neurotoxin injection every 4 months. My goal is for my outside to match how I feel on the inside.

I quote this study to make a point. People struggle with issues or occurrences in their lives that looking better will not fully resolve (nor will alcohol, drugs, gambling, sex, eating, not eating or a shopping addiction for that matter). Listen, if I am going to call myself a 'good doctor,' I certainly am going to have to look at my patient as a fellow human being and not just a 'face.'

I am fortunate to have an arsenal of skin care ingredients and medical aesthetic procedures to employ in an attempt to make someone look and feel more youthful. It is important, however, to illustrate what these procedures *won't* do. Skin care and medical aesthetic professionals need to be aware that a client is an entire person. As a patient visiting a cosmetic physician/medical spa, it is important to convey this as well.

What Botox Won't Do

1. Botox Won't Get Your X back

I saw a case report of a woman whose boyfriend left her. The next thing she did was to walk into a plastic surgeon's office with a picture of Jessica Alba and announced to the doctor, "Make me look like her." Since her boyfriend had a fondness for Jessica Alba, the woman was willing to go to any lengths to look like her in an attempt to get him back. While this is certainly an extreme case, it is quite believable.

The surgeon operated on her face, I suspect after reviewing the '*no guarantee the boyfriend would return*' disclaimer. This is certainly a disturbing example; however, I've had plenty of men and women desiring a treatment with the goal of finding a date. Medical aesthetic offices are no stranger to single moms and dads. So while I most certainly can make you look and feel more youthful, I can't fix a broken relationship.

However, I have no problem discussing other options with clients about how to cope with feelings of loneliness and perhaps connect them up with a good psychologist if they are willing. Do I do this with everyone on the dating scene? No, but if it seems to control the majority of the conversation during the visit, my need to interject other options is far more likely.

2.   Get You A Job

I have attempted to help people with this goal many times. In a perfect world employers would care only about people's credentials and the ability to perform the job well. Alas, it is not a perfect world. I experienced this with my own father. He was in the insurance industry and worked diligently at the same company for over 20 years. When it closed, he couldn't find a job. Although he was only in his late forties, he looked older than his age and was up against fresh young faces. People who are considered attractive also make more money than their less attractive counterparts. That's reality. So while I can't get you a job I certainly can help you look and feel the very best before that next interview

3.   Cure Your Depression

25% of the population suffers from some form of anxiety or depression. So if I treat 12 people in a day, the odds are that 3 of them are dealing with this issue at some level. I am aware of this. Every doctor or health care professional should be thinking about it as well.

4.   Get You Through a Mid-Life Crisis

The average age of my clients historically has been between 35-55 years of age. A mid-life crisis could defined as, *"An emotional crisis of identity and self-confidence that can occur in early middle age."* Women around the age of 50 get another whammy with menopause thrown into the mix. I can help you look and feel younger but there are many others out there including psychiatrists, psychologists, therapists and your primary care MD that can help you through these troubling years.

5. Botox Won't Change Your Lifestyle

While the procedures I perform may only take 30-60 minutes and I can recommend the best skin care regimen for you, the rest is up to you and I have a few skin saving guidelines:

- **Stay out of the sun** – sunbathing feels great but it is a collagen killer, age spot maker and can cause skin cancer. I realize I discuss this quite a bit, perhaps I am reminding myself at some level. I have loved the sun through the years far too much and my skin has definitely suffered.

- **Take it easy on the sugar** – Foods with a high glycemic load can cause a rise in blood glucose and insulin levels. When your body absorbs sugars quickly, the pancreas secretes insulin in response. A spike in insulin can lead to a spike in hormone levels. This affects both the circulation to your skin and the rate of turnover of newer vibrant cells. Lots of sugar = dull complexion.

- **Stop scrubbing your skin** – excessive use of harsh cleansers, aggressive brushing or heaven forbid a loofah will strip your skin of its protective oils and lead to a dry and less radiant complexion. Use a gentle cleanser and wash with your fingertips. If using a rotating or sonic exfoliating brush, easy does it.

- **Get enough sleep** – Most people under 60 need 7-8 hours of sleep to look and feel their best. Stay away from caffeine, TV and computers at night as they are all far too stimulating to be used before you are attempting to sleep. Chamomile Tea is helpful to many. Alcohol in moderation.

- **Drink four-five 16oz glasses of water/day** – This has been mentioned with the Clear Skin diet. Wellness can be a daunting venture to many. Any fear you have about wellness or living a healthy lifestyle, by and large is unwarranted. I didn't always drink enough water. I knew I should drink more. Finally one day I put a 16oz plastic glass on the counter and filled it at least 4 times. Making a decision doesn't need to take months or years. Just do it.

Case Study: I had a 46 year old woman in my office one January morning. She came in about every 4 months for Botox. This day she was 'dead set' on her New Year resolution to lose weight and live a healthy lifestyle. She was 5'4 and 145#. I talked with her about ideal weight, diet and exercise. I knew her though. She had this same resolution the year before. I told her that if she kept in touch with me and followed my **three** recommendations for 4 months, her next Botox treatment would be free. My three recommendations were:

1. Drink no less than 64 ounces of water every day and preferably a significant portion of those ounces before meals.
2. Take a 30 minute walk every other day. Walk briskly enough that you feel a tad winded but certainly can continue without resting (i.e. fat burn).
3. With every meal replace 8 ounces of what she would normally eat with an 8 ounce portion of antioxidant-rich vegetables from the Clear Skin diet. As a reminder: Arugula, Kale, Collard Greens, Brussel Sprouts, Chard, Romaine Lettuce and spinach.

We traded emails over the course of the next four months and she called and spoke with my staff several times. She was sticking with this *simple* plan. When she returned in May she was more than ready for summer. She had lost 12 pounds and her skin had never looked better. She looked years younger. Her explanation was one I have heard before. "I felt *so much better* after walking 30 minutes every-other-day, after a few weeks I just started walking *every day.*" It turns out that she likes spinach and drinking water before meals essentially kept her skin hydrated and made her less hungry. A simple plan always works better than a complicated one.

- **Exercise in moderation**

The case study above demonstrated how healthy moderate exercise is for you. Exercise increases blood flow to the skin. It also aids in the clearance of cellular waste products including free radicals. Those that exercise regularly sleep better too.

In my 20+ years in practice I have seen changes in the world around us and people seem increasingly stressed out. Stress is no good for anyone's health, including their skin health. While I continually strive to help others to look and feel their best, sometimes our busy world and life takes its toll. That is when it is time to lean on others who can help you while doing certain *simple things* that will assure you age gracefully … and beautifully.

Comparing the Neurotoxins

Botox's seven year run as America's only cosmetic neurotoxin ended abruptly in 2009 with the arrival of Dysport (abobotulinum toxin A; approved in other countries since 1991). Botox now had a legitimate challenger in the US marketplace. Next in line was Xeomin (**Zee**-Oh-Min). It had been used in Europe since 2008 and received FDA approval in November of 2011 making it the newest neurotoxin on the US market.

Neurotoxin	Botox Cosmetic	Dysport	Xeomin
Generic Name	Onabotulinum Toxin A	Abobotulinum Toxin A	Incobotulinum Toxin A
Benefits and	Trusted Brand	Works Faster	No Refrigeration
Claimed benefits *	Highly Researched	Lasts Longer*	Less Expensive*

Dysport

Seemingly, treating one side of the face with Botox and the other side with Dysport would make for a pretty compelling study. A plastic surgeon from San Francisco thought so as well. In 2011 he performed a "Split Face" study of 90 patients comparing the effectiveness of Botox vs. Dysport. He focused on one area, the crow's feet (technically known as 'the lateral orbital rhytids). The patients were asked to evaluate their satisfaction with each side using a 5-point scale. Two-thirds of the participants preferred the Dysport side. Neither the researchers nor the patients knew which side received which treatment (double-blind study).

On initial appearances it seemed like a slam dunk win for Dysport. But wait, the study was financed by Medicis (the makers of Dysport) and the researchers used a 3:1 ratio of Dysport to Botox.

Technically anywhere from **2.5-3.0** units of Dysport are considered to be the equivalent of 1 unit of Botox. Was the deck stacked in Dysport's favor? Allergan (the maker of Botox) said the difference in score between the products was negligible, just 0.2 points on the 5-point scale. Allergan said, "It's unlikely this difference is relevant in terms of patients' results." They added this was certainly "not grounds to base a claim of superiority."

I am Not Quick to Change what Works

I was resistant to use Dysport initially. I had been very comfortable using Botox and enjoyed its dosing and predictable results. The introduction of a new product seemed like an unwanted nuisance. I was not alone. Many of my colleagues shared my hesitancy. Dysport is associated with a smaller protein which means it can spread out more than Botox after injection. This is both good and bad news. If I am injecting large areas such as the forehead or under the arms to reduce sweating that means fewer injection sites using Dysport; a clear advantage when it comes to patient comfort. But what about the small muscles in the brow or around the eyes? Do I want a lot of diffusion there along with an increased risk of side effects like a teary eye or droopy lid? As is the case in the *practice* of medicine, I knew what I needed to do; *practice* and learn how to use Dysport safely and effectively.

This brings up a very important point. When new neurotoxins or other medical aesthetic treatments enter the marketplace, many professionals are quick to offer them. It always makes an office look 'cutting edge' to have the newest treatments available. Do your homework and make sure whoever you are seeing has had adequate training with the new injection or procedure.

My Opinion: Dysport Does Have an Advantage

My experience, supported by the literature, is that Dysport appears to have a faster onset of action than Botox. If you need a quick fix for a wedding or upcoming event 1-3 days away, Dysport may be a better option with an onset of action of 1-3 days vs. Botox's 3-5 days. On occasion there is a patient who becomes 'resistant' to Botox after extended use. This is not a common occurrence. On these rare occasions, this person would be an excellent candidate for Dysport.

Cost is another consideration. Prior to coming to the US, the prices for Dysport in the UK were less per treatment area than Botox. In the US, understanding that you need about 2.5-3.0 units of Dysport per 1.0 unit of Botox, prices for Dysport are typically in the range of $4-6/unit with Botox selling for $10-15/unit. Hence, in offices that offer both the cost difference per area treated is negligible.

Side Effects

The most important factor when choosing where to get Botox or Dysport is the clinical ability and experience of the person doing the injections. Let me say that again. The best treatment is not the cheapest or newest treatment, it is the treatment given by a well-trained and experienced injector. I give people an option as to which neurotoxin they wish to choose along with a conversation about how many years I have been injecting Botox vs. Dysport and potential side effects. After administering thousands of injections of these two neurotoxins, by far the most common side effect I have seen is bruising at the injection site. Others include eye irritation, watery eye, light sensitivity and eyelid drooping. Choose wisely and find out how long your injector has been at it.

Competition is good for Consumers

With competition in the marketplace, this means you are more likely to find promotions and rebates from Allergen (Botox) and Medicis (Dysport). They both want your business and your loyalty. I am comfortable injecting either. In the big picture, they are nearly equivalent in terms of what they do to reduce fine lines and wrinkles. Dysport gets the nod for a quicker onset. My experience is that Dysport and Botox last about the same amount of time (3-4 months).

Xeomin

Xeomin from Merz Aesthetics has been used in Europe since 2008. It received FDA approval in November of 2011 and is the newest neurotoxin on the US market. However, Xeomin (inco-botulinumtoxinA) did not come out of the gate smoothly. It was pulled in March of 2012 following a federal court ruling that Merz collected consumer lists and sales figures from Allergan (the maker of Botox). The confidential information was obtained through Allergan sales representatives. So after a rocky start, Xeomin was re-launched in early 2013.

Botox and Xeomin are very similar. Xeomin is sometimes described as "The Naked Botox." This is because while Botox has carrier proteins, Xeomin does not and hence is 'naked.' In theory this absence of protein carriers results in fewer allergic reactions or resistance to the neurotoxin. Xeomin, due to its lack of these additives, does not need to be refrigerated. It is the only one of the three neurotoxins that has this feature. As we will see, the fact that Xeomin does not need to be refrigerated is indeed a benefit.

Xeomin 'Advantages'

1. *In theory*, less people will develop resistance via antibody formation. If you have a cold, the body makes antibodies to fight off that virus. When that virus comes around again, the antibodies quickly neutralize it. Hence, the body is *resistant.*

The human body doesn't commonly make antibodies to Botox. In the small percentage that do, the effect and duration of action of Botox are markedly reduced. In the very few patients I have seen with this resistance, I switch to Dysport. Xeomin could be another alternative to Botox in this situation.

2. *In theory*, fewer allergic reactions. Merz aesthetics attributes this to the absence of carrier proteins as well. After injecting Botox for over 10 years I can honestly say I have never experienced a patient allergy to Botox. James Bonaparte, MD, Cosmetic Surgeon and researcher would seem to agree as he notes, "After reviewing 20,000 patients and a number of randomized studies, there are no reports of allergies with Botox."

3. No refrigeration needed. Botox and Dysport are shipped in dry ice. Hence, Xeomin is cheaper to ship and adds a measure of convenience here.

Onset and Duration of Action:

Botox and Xeomin are essentially identical in terms of the active neurotoxin ingredient. One unit of Botox = One unit of Xeomin. (One unit of Botox = 2.5 Units of Dysport). Thus the conversion is simple. If you had a good result to your brow with 20 units of Botox, you should get the same result with 20 units of Xeomin (or 50 units of Dysport).

Dysport clearly has a faster onset of action than Botox. (1-3 days vs. 3-5 days *on average)*. Xeomin's 3-5 day onset of action mirrors Botox. There are case reports stating Xeomin works faster, however there is no proof behind these claims. Certainly if such a study existed, Merz Aesthetics would have let us know. Equally common are reports of Xeomin being cheaper because it 'doesn't last as long.' There is no study supporting this either.

Xeomin and Botox both will last 3-4 months. Results vary person to person and are affected by factors such as activity level, amount injected and area injected.

Cost

Xeomin may cost the doctor less than Botox depending on how much he/she is buying (up to 15% less). Whether or not they pass the savings along to you depends on each individual practice. Many offices, to simplify matters, charge the same per-unit price for Botox and Xeomin. Based on the practices I reviewed, the average for Botox is $12-$14/unit and Xeomin $9-12/unit. Overall the average savings is $1-2 per unit of Xeomin (vs Botox). Merz Aesthetics has offered different promotions in the past, such as a $50 gift card when 30 units or more of Xeomin were purchased.

Having three products instead of one is good for consumers as each company is vying for your business and your loyalty. Through rebates, gift cards and award programs, many discounts are available as each company wants you using their product and is willing to reward you for doing so.

Trusted Brands

Products like Coca-Cola, Heinz, Kleenex, Viagra, and Botox have had great success along with names that bring forth a clear image to consumers. They are known and trusted brands. There are other colas, catsups, tissues, erectile dysfunction medications and neurotoxins, but if someone says "Botox", the vast majority of the population knows exactly what you are talking about. It's the gold standard; the tried and true neurotoxin used a long time while giving consistent, safe and predictable results. Dysport was called "The new Botox" and Xeomin has been called "The naked Botox." Even competitors are described in 'Botox' terms. **Botox** is a strong, enduring and trusted brand.

The Xeomin Verdict

The most tangible benefits to recommend Xeomin are firstly, its slightly lower cost (*in some offices*), and secondly, the fact that it does not need to be refrigerated. The theories that it will cause less resistance or allergies are not likely to make one shred of difference in the success or failure of Xeomin.

As it stands in 2016, Botox is to medical aesthetics as Coca-Cola is to soft drinks. Time will tell how Xeomin will fit in as a player in the neurotoxin market. The fact that it really does not have a glaring downside is important. I certainly feel it is an effective and worthy neurotoxin to use as an alternative to Botox or Dysport.

The Future of Neurotoxins

When I first began studying and practicing medical aesthetics there was only Botox in the US. Then came Dysport came, followed quickly by Xeomin. My feeling is that Xeomin will not be the last. If dermal fillers (discussed in the next chapter) are any indication, more neurotoxins are forthcoming.

However, there is something that could bring and abrupt halt to the injectable neurotoxin market. In fact, injectable neurotoxins may be well on their way to becoming obsolete. Nobody stays on top for ever, even Botox.

Botox binds to facial nerves to ultimately prevent contraction of facial muscles. A type of peptide known as a *Neuropeptide* (specifically Argeline) has been shown to block chemicals involved with nerve innervation. Once these neuropeptides are able to be applied to the skin and be absorbed to the nerve, there will be a shift in the world of neurotoxins and the roles of injectable neurotoxins such as Botox. Time will tell.

Chapter Seven

Dermal Fillers

I had a 34 year old client in my office, joined by her friend. As my client was getting prepped for a dermal filler injection, her friend proudly announced, "I have been very fortunate to have perfect skin and no wrinkles." While her comment was a bit off-putting, she was actually right. Although she and my client were of similar age, this woman's skin was indeed quite flawless. She never had any medical aesthetic or surgical procedure and did very little in regard to skin care. I like to refer to this small group of the population as those that *hit the genetics lottery.* The vast majority of people need a little help. Dermal fillers come to the rescue in a big way.

Dermal fillers are the #2 most sought after and administered medical aesthetic treatment. Botox may have a topical preparation lurking and potentially replacing it. Dermal fillers are here to stay. It has now been over a decade since Restylane was FDA approved (March, 2005) and it would appear as though Ellanse will be the next dermal filler to hit the US marketplace. Dermal fillers are *very* popular. The reason is simple. They offer a safe and effective way to bring youthful results without expensive cosmetic surgery. Most patients who have had dermal fillers are happy and come back for more.

However, with the arrival of new dermal fillers and different formulations it can be difficult to determine which filler works best for each 'wrinkle.' Dermal fillers are approved by the FDA for treatment of specific areas of the face. Radiesse was approved by the FDA for treatment of naso-labial folds back in 2006. Nine years later in 2015 it received an approval for "improvement of volume loss on the dorsum (back) of the hands." Dermal fillers are FDA approved for certain areas with other uses designated as 'off label' uses.

The FDA and Off Label Uses

Back in December of 2003, Restylane became the first hyaluronic acid dermal filler FDA approved for correction of volume loss in the naso-labial folds. Since that time, an estimated 18 million procedures with Restylane have been performed. Restylane would not be alone for long. Soon we saw Hylaform Sculptra, Captique, Juvederm, Artefill, Elevess, Radiesse, Prevelle and Belotero along with 18 more FDA approved uses.

In regard to 'off label' uses of dermal fillers; There is nothing wrong with a doctor injecting into an area other than the FDA approved area. Mark Jewell, MD, author of *Safety with Injectables Workbook* agrees. He says, "Off-label use is legitimate, it's something a doctor discusses with the patient to meet the patient's specific needs."

So provided the injector is experienced and the doctor and patient are in agreement, there is no problem injecting into areas that are 'off label.' It is important to note, however, that *advertising injections* into off-label areas is not considered to be acceptable.

Dermal fillers injection results are very injector-dependent. There is no other area of medical aesthetics where the experience, technique and artistic ability of the doctor, nurse or medical aesthetician are more important. Obtaining a beautiful and natural result has more to do with the ability of the injector than which filler is injected. Dermal filler injection is the most artistic realm of medical aesthetics. It has always been my favorite part of the practice of medical aesthetics.

Understanding Dermal Fillers

Certain factors need to be understood to deterine why certain fillers work better in a given area of the face. These include the primary ingredients, cross-linking, particle size, concentration and G-prime.

Primary Ingredients

Primary ingredients are essentially what the dermal filler is 'made of.' The vast majority of dermal fillers are composed of hyaluronic acid.

1.   Hyaluronic Acid

Hyaluronic acid is a natural substance found in body tissues. It is a glycosaminoglycan that is present in the highest concentrations in connective tissue, cartilage, joint fluids and the skin. Hyaluronic acid fillers are a clear gel on appearance. A huge benefit of these fillers is their ability to draw water to themselves. This helps to increase the longevity of the filler. In individuals that remain well hydrated these fillers have a tendency to last an extra month or more. Dermal fillers composed of hyaluronic acid include Restylane, Juvederm, Belotero, Elevess, Prevelle, and Evolence.

2.   Calcium Hydroxylapatite

Calcium hydroxylapatite is a mineral-like substance found in human bone. It is the heaviest of all dermal fillers. While hyaluronic acid fillers are clear in appearance, calcium hydroxylapatite appears milky white. A benefit of this type of dermal filler is its ability to powerfully stimulate collagen formation. Radiesse is an example of this type of dermal filler.

3.   Poly-L-Lactic Acid (PLLA)

PLLA is a synthetic dermal filler that is injected 'throughout' the face. In doing so (similar to Radiesse) it stimulates the production of collagen. PLLA is different from other fillers in that it does not produce immediate results. Rather, through the stimulation of collagen formation in the dermis, the results appear gradually over several months. Sculptra is the only FDA approved PLLA dermal filler.

4. Polymethyl-Methacrylate (PMMA)

PMMA fillers are composed of PMMA microspheres suspended in purified collagen gel. Months following injection the gel breaks down and is replaced by your body's own collagen. This is commonly (and incorrectly) referred to as 'semi-permanent.' The PMMA is not fully metabolized so some remains in the skin permanently. An example of this filler is Bellafill. It is associated with lumps, nodules, granulomas and requires many injections. There are those who are very fond of PMMA fillers. I am not one of them. I do not recommend them. There are far better options.

Cross Linking

In the discussion of hyaluronic acid fillers, cross-linking is of particular interest. The natural liquid form of hyaluronic acid is quickly metabolized by the body in less than 24 hours. Cross-linking transforms the liquid form of hyaluronic acid to a gel form. This cross-linking dramatically slows the body's ability to metabolize the hyaluronic acid. Hence, the cross-linked hyaluronic acid fillers will last many months. Dermal fillers with more cross-linking of hyaluronic acid generally last longer.

Particle Size and Concentration

As a general rule, dermal fillers with higher concentrations and larger particle sizes tend to be better suited for injection more deeply beneath the skin surface. A dermal filler with a higher concentration is *typically* felt to last longer. For instance, Restylane has a concentration of 20mg/ml while Juvederm Ultra's is 24mg/ml. On first appearance, it would appear as though Juvederm would last longer due to the higher concentration. However, Restylane's syringe is larger at 1.0 ml vs. Juvederm Ultra's 0.8 ml. Hence, they both last about the same amount of time.

Dermal filler concentration is commonly described as 'particles per ml.' More particles per ml equates to a smaller particle size. Larger particles tend to last longer and are better for deeper injection. As an example, in terms of particle concentration, Restylane's is 100,000/ml, Restylane Lyft's is 10,000/ml and Restylane Silk's is 500,000/ml. The larger particle size makes Restylane Lyft a better choice for deeper injection while Silk would be preferable for a more superficial injection to delicate areas.

Filler	Particles /ml	Particle Size	Best areas to inject:
Restylane Silk	500,000	Small	Superficial/ delicate
Restylane	100,000	Medium	Multiple areas
Restylane Lyft	10,000	Large	Deeper dermis (and below)
Juvederm Voluma	Variable	Variable	Deep dermis (and below)

Juvederm Voluma is used for deeper injections. Voluma demonstrates that large particle size is not necessarily synonymous with deep injection. Its particle sizes are 'variable' and as we find out later in this chapter, most are of a smaller size.

G-Prime

Dermal fillers with a higher G-prime are thicker, heavier and 'harder.' They are more resistant to disintegration however may also be more painful to the patient during injection. Dermal fillers with a higher G-prime are typically injected deeper into the dermis. They are better suited for injection into deeper folds such as the nasolabial fold or to increase cheek or face volume.

I prefer fillers with a higher G-prime when I desire a 'lifting' effect in the cheek area. A lifting effect means the dermal filler has the ability to literally *PULL the area UP*. It is important to note, however, that simply having a higher G-prime does not necessarily equate to a product with a better 'lifting effect.' A product such as Juvederm Voluma has a G-prime lower than other dermal fillers yet has an excellent lifting effect. In truth, the lifting effect involves several factors including G-prime, concentration, and ability of the filler to intercollege (or 'grab') surrounding tissues. Examples of higher G-prime fillers include Radiesse and Restylane Lyft. Dermal fillers with a lower G-prime are thinner and lighter. They are better suited for injection into delicate areas such as the tear troughs, lips or other superficial wrinkles. Examples of this type of filler include Restylane Silk, Belotero and Prevelle.

The Tyndall Effect

This is an effect that can occur with some hyaluronic acid fillers when injected superficially. This effect is the result of light reflecting off of the filler (beneath the skin) giving a bluish hue. We know hyaluronic fillers all have distinct cross-linking, concentrations, particle sizes and G-primes. Fillers with more cross-linking and a higher G-prime are better suited for deeper injections to add more volume. They are *also* more likely to produce a Tyndall effect thus should not be injected superficially.

Belotero boasts that its low G-prime and variable cross-linking attributes make it stand alone as the only filler that can be injected superficially and never result in a Tyndall effect. The presence of the Tyndall effect is something exceedingly rare in my experience. The likelihood of this effect occurring increases the more superficially the filler is placed. I have seen case reports of these occurrences. In most cases it appears as though the filler was placed at the top of the dermis or even intra-epidermally (i.e. *barely* beneath the skin surface). Essentially any filler injected very superficially may result in this effect.

All these features of dermal fillers can indeed get confusing. Essentially, dermal fillers with larger particles, higher concentrations, a higher G-prime and more extensive cross-linking tend to last longer, be bulkier, 'stickier,' add more volume, and are better suited for deeper injection into the dermis. For fine and delicate and more superficial injection, fillers with a smaller particle size, lower concentration, less crosslinking and a lower G-prime are preferable. Based on these factors the guide on the following page gives you my preference for which dermal filler ideally should be placed where. The choice of dermal filler relies heavily on the discussion between the patient and injector each's preference and/or experience. Some dermal fillers shouldn't be placed in certain areas. For example, the consistency of Radiesse makes it an excellent choice for cheek augmentation but a terrible choice for lips.

Dermal Filler Property	Best for superficial injection (delicate areas)	Best for Deeper injection (more volume)	Best for "Lifting Effect"
G-Prime	Lower	higher	higher
Concentration & particle size	More particles/ml	Fewer particles/ml	Fewer particles/ml
	(=smaller particles)	(=larger particles)	(=larger particles)

DERMAL FILLER GUIDE

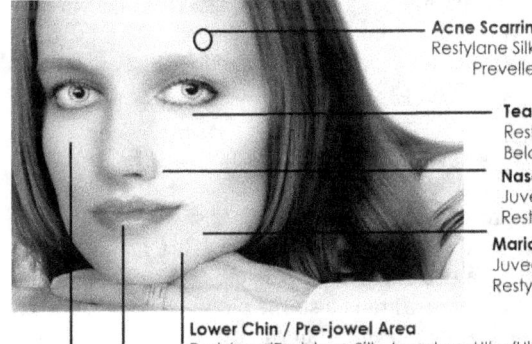

Acne Scarring (anywhere)
Restylane Silk, Belotero, Prevelle Silk

Tear Troughs
Restylane/Restylane Silk, Belotero

Naso-Labial Folds
Juvederm Ultra/Ultra Plus, Restylane, Radiesse

Marionette Lines
Juvederm Ultra/Ultra Plus, Restylane, Radiesse

Lower Chin / Pre-jowel Area
Restylane/Restylane Silk, Juvederm Ultra/Ultra Plus, Belotero

Lips and Lip Lines (smoker's lines)
Restylane/ Restylane Silk, Juvederm Ultra, Belotero

Cheek Augmentation
Radiesse, Juvederm Voluma, Restylane Lyft

Dermal Filler Options

Before discussing each of the dermal fillers, it is important to first discuss injection techniques. People spend a great deal of time worrying about which filler is best or which is most cost-effective. The fact is that dermal filler results are injector-dependent. Suppose you have determined that you would like to have a dermal filler injection to your naso-labial folds with Restylane. The injector takes the needle filled with 1.0 ml of the product and quickly injects the full contents of the syringe into each naso-labial fold. It would seem on the surface to be perhaps exactly what should have been done. However, the injector's technique was terrible.

Dermal filler injection is an art. Two things need to be accomplished with the injection. Think of it like this: First, I am putting a needle into the dermis which is filled with collagen-making fibroblasts. Second, I want the dermal filler to be spread out so there is more surface area present. Through accomplishing this, the filler has a better ability to do its 'work'. If it is a hyaluronic acid filler, that means drawing more moisture to it. If it's Radiesse, it means more surface area is present to stimulate collagen growth.

Another advantage of putting the filler in and 'fanning out' the product is that through multiple short, gentle passages, that needle will do wonders for stimulating more collagen. Dermal filler attributes are important but injector technique holds the key to a great result.

Juvederm Ultra

In 2010 Juvederm Ultra was FDA approved to last 'up to a year.' I read a case report of a woman who had Juvederm Ultra in her lips for a year and a half and wanted it removed because it just wouldn't go away. That is rare. Juvederm Ultra is a sterile gel made up of crossed linked hyaluronic acid. I have been a fan of Juvederm Ultra but my experience is that it lasts closer to 5-6 months, occasionally longer. It really depends on the area injected. Also, some people just break down the product faster than others. Areas around the mouth and lips have more movement and tend to have a shorter life-span for dermal fillers. The naso-labial folds last longer. Juvederm has a very smooth consistency making it quite popular and very versatile. It can be used effectively in many areas of the face. I recommend its use for naso-labial folds, lips, marionette lines and peri-oral lines.

Juvederm Ultra Plus

Juvederm Ultra Plus contains hyaluronic acid molecules of a much larger size than Juvederm Ultra. The filler itself is denser and thicker with more cross-linking. Due to these characteristics, Juvederm Ultra Plus is beneficial for deeper injections and adds more volume than Juvederm Ultra. It also lasts longer. As you may imagine, Juvederm Ultra Plus also is more expensive than Juvederm Ultra. This product works very well in the naso-labial and marionette line areas. While it can also be used for cheek augmentation, Juvederm Voluma is much superior in this regard.

Juvederm Voluma

Allergan has been at the forefront of medical aesthetics with products such as Botox Cosmetic and Juvederm for over a decade. Juvederm Ultra has had tremendous success but one common complaint was the lack of duration of the filler. Much like Restylane, the filler doesn't typically last longer than 6 months. Juvederm Ultra Plus in many cases lasts much longer, even up to a year with an average of 6-9 months.

At the 11th Congress of Anti-Aging and Aesthetic Medicine in Monaco, Allergan unveiled the Vycross Technology present in Juvederm Voluma (and Volbella / Volift). Most hyaluronic acid fillers are made with cross linked 100% high molecular weight hyaluronic acid. With Vycross technology these fillers are made with only 10% high molecular weight and 90% low molecular weight hyaluronic acid. The cross linking between the variable size hyaluronic acid molecules results in a filler that lasts much longer and brings other favorable results.

Juvederm Voluma, despite its lower G-Prime brings a superior lifting effect. The old notion that only high G-prime fillers can bring 'lift' has clearly been proven wrong with Juvederm Voluma. My experience is that the variable molecular sizes and cross-linking of hyaluronic acid molecules present with Voluma allows for the filler's ability to 'grab' onto surrounding tissues. In the 4/1/2014 issue of the

Dermatology Times, Vic Narurkar, MD noted, "The ability to intercollate gives Voluma its ability to lift … It lifts better than any of the fillers currently approved by the FDA."

In the USA, Juvederm Voluma broke new ground as well when it became the first dermal filler with the indication "for deep injection *for cheek augmentation* to correct age-related volume deficit in the mid-face in adults over the age of 21."

Benefits of Juvederm Voluma

- The filler is very smooth which makes the injection less painful to the patient.

- There is typically less swelling after injection.

- Patients have been satisfied with the 'natural' results.

Does it last 2 years?

Allergan bases its claim of the (up to) 2 year longevity of its filler based on a study where 6-8 mls of Voluma was injected into the cheeks of subjects. After two years the participants were asked if they felt the product was still present. A 'yes' meant they answered 1 or above on a scale of 1-6. The volume injected was intended to reflect a 'full correction.'

The only issue I have with this study is the amount that was injected. It is exceedingly rare that I inject this much filler into a patient in a single appointment. Most experts agree that Juvederm Voluma lasts 18 months or more. Despite the issue I have with the amount injected, the same appears to hold true when smaller amounts are injected. And really … who can blame the company (Allergan) for injecting lots of it to help prove their point? It is my opinion that Juvederm Voluma is a very effective dermal filler. It is excellent for face volumization and brings a solid lifting effect in the cheeks. While Juvederm Voluma is FDA approved in the US, Juvederm Volbella and Volift are not. However, these are used just about everywhere else including Canada, Europe and Mexico.

- Juvederm Voluma - Best used for restoration of volume loss in the face / cheeks

- Juvederm Volbella - Best used for adding fullness to lips and fine lines around the lips

- Juvederm Volift – Most effective to areas such as naso-labial folds and marionette lines.

I have been a fan of Radiesse (discussed later in this chapter) for volumization of the cheeks for many years. I am aware that times change and technology improves. I will say that while I have had excellent results with Radiesse, Juvederm Voluma offers a worthy alternative.

The Restylane Family

At the time of this writing, it has been nearly 13 years since Restylane received its first FDA approval for "*Injection into the mid to deep dermis for correction of moderate to severe facial wrinkles and folds (such as nasolabial folds)."* That approval came 12/12/2003. Since that time, Restylane has been a go-to hyaluronic acid dermal filler for many medical aesthetic doctors and cosmetic surgeons. It was the first hyaluronic filler on the market and has been used an estimated 15 million times. In the past five years, hyaluronic acid filler injections have nearly doubled in popularity (a 94% increase).

'Restylane' is the trade name for the hyaluronic acid filler which has been manufactured by Q-Med, Medicis, Valeant and Galderma. These companies have been busy with the FDA over the past 12 years gaining new indications thus keeping Restylane a strong option for injection to just about any area of the face. There are new products being developed and introduced at an increasing rate all vying for a place in the growing medical aesthetic arena. Restylane of recent years has actually been gaining momentum with four new indications in the past four years.

Restylane Type	Approval Date	Indication
Restylane Lyft (formerly Perlane)	7/1/2015	Moderate to severe facial folds and wrinkles in patients over the age of 21 who have age-related volume loss.
Restylane Silk	6/13/2014	Indicated for lip augmentation and dermal implantation for correction of peri-oral rhytids (wrinkles around the lips) in patients 21 and up.
Restylane - L	8/30/2012	Injection into the mid to deep dermis for correction of moderate to severe facial wrinkles/folds (such as naso-labial folds) **and** for lip augmentation in patients 21 and up.
Restylane	10/11/2011	Lip augmentation in those over 21 years of age.

Source: FDA.gov

As it stands today there are four types of Restylane. These include Restylane, Restylane-L, Restylane Silk, and Restylane Lyft.

Restylane

Like Juvederm, Restylane is a sterile gel made up of crossed-linked hyaluronic acid. Restylane and Juvederm are popular because they work well and have strong safety profiles. Restylane's cross-linked hyaluronic acid is smaller in size than that of Juvederm Ultra. This allows for better use in more delicate areas such as around the eyes, tear troughs, around the lips and "frown lines" between the eyebrows. Many times when trying to determine which filler is best it comes down to patient experience. If a patient had Juvederm Ultra in her lips or naso-labial folds and it lasted nearly a year, the best bet is to try it again. Restylane, like Juvederm Ultra lasts for 5-6 months and tends to be more modestly priced than other fillers.

<u>Restylane – L</u>

This is simply regular Restylane pre-mixed with lidocaine

<u>Restylane Silk</u>

Restylane Silk is a hyaluronic acid filler consisting of smoother and smaller particles than Restylane. Restylane Silk's small size (500,000/ml) and ultra-smooth consistency gained it FDA approval for fine lines around the mouth as well as lip augmentation. It is also an excellent choice for tear troughs and filling in deeper acne scars.

<u>Restylane Lyft</u>

Restlane Lyft was previously known as 'Perlane.' It has always been a favorite of mine for injection of the naso-labial folds, marionette lines and for cheek augmentation. It has the largest particle size at 10,000/ml. Restylane Lyft is FDA approved for, "*moderate to severe facial folds and wrinkles and age related volume loss*." Restylane Lyft is an excellent filler for injection into the naso-labial folds, marionette lines and for cheek augmentation. Restylane Lyft, Juvederm Voluma and Radiesse offer the best 'lift' to the cheek area of all available fillers.

Prevelle

Prevelle was FDA approved in 2008 and has been used worldwide. Prevelle Silk is simply Prevelle *plus lidocaine*. It is not as commonly used as Restylane or Juvederm but there is indeed a place for it. Prevelle is at the opposite end of the spectrum from products such as Restylane Lyft or Radiesse. It has a *low molecular weight* and is the smallest molecule in this class. Prevelle's best use may be as an entry level dermal filler. With someone who is new to dermal fillers or hesitant to make big changes, Prevelle is an excellent choice. It tends to cause less swelling and is best used for fine lines and wrinkles as well as for lip augmentation. The downside with Prevelle is that it just doesn't seem to last very long; typically 3-4 months. The upside is that it is less expensive and if someone is hesitant and/or looking for subtle changes to the naso-labial folds, around the mouth, tear troughs or lips, Prevelle may be a good option. Those I have injected with Prevelle tended to not want dramatic changes and were pleased with the lower cost.

Radiesse

Radiesse's composition is calicium hydroxylapatite (a constituent of bone and cartilage). Unlike hyaluronic acid fillers that appear clear in the syringe, Radiesse has a milky-white consistency. Being thicker allows Radiesse to do a few things perhaps better than the hyaluronic acid fillers. I like to use Radiesse for cheek augmentation. It is very robust. When injected into the cheek or mid-face it offers an excellent volumizing and lifting effect. In addition, Radiesse stimulates new collagen. Radiesse can also be used to for naso-labial folds or marionette lines. It is a bit more expensive ($700-900 per syringe) however comes as a 1.5 ml syringe (vs. 1.0 with Restylane). Radiesse lasts longer too, typically 12-18 months in most patients.

Sculptra

Sculptra is a collagen stimulator and is really in its own class. It continues to gain momentum in the US however it is really nothing new at all. The original formulation was used in Europe since 1999. It is composed of Poly-L-Lactic-Acid (PLLA). While it is classified as a dermal filler it works much differently than the others. After the filler is injected it strongly stimulates collagen while the Sculptra itself is slowly absorbed.

Sculptra is injected *throughout* the face. It has been described as very beneficial at filling in 'grooves and hollows' due to volume loss. It works particularly well in those with volume loss in areas such as the cheeks, temples or jawline. It also adds volume beautifully in other more commonly injected areas such as the naso-labial folds and marionette lines. Sculptra should not be used in the brow, forehead or around the eyes, mouth or lips.

The injections are completed in a series of sessions 6 weeks apart. It works very slowly taking up to six months to demonstrate its full effect. Done correctly the results are very natural and subtle. Sculptra has been used to correct the facial tissue loss genetic to certain families or that seen with HIV patients. Also, when the health of the patient precludes plastic surgery, Sculptra is strong alternative.

Belotero

Belotero was introduced to the UK in January, 2007. Like most other medical aesthetic treatments, the US had to wait; in this case nearly 5 years until Belotero was finally approved in November of 2011. The FDA approval was for *injection into facial tissue to smooth wrinkles and folds especially around the nose and mouth (naso-labial folds).* Belotero is a hyaluronic acid filler. It entered the market in competition with other hyaluronic acid fillers such as Juvederm (ultra, ultra plus and voluma), Restylane, Restylane Silk and Prevelle Silk.

There are 3 types of Belotero, only one (Belotero Balance) is approved in the US.

1. **Belotero Balance** (previously known as Belotero 'Basic') – This has an 'average' concentration of hyaluronic acid (22.5mg/ml), with a wide array of uses including naso-labial folds, marionette lines, lips, brow lines and crow's feet.

2. **Belotero Soft** – Has a slightly lower concentration (20mg/ml). It comes with a smaller needle (30g) which makes it ideal for injection to superficial wrinkles, lips, crow's feet and forehead wrinkles. This is injected more superficially, into the upper dermis, than Belotero Intense which would is injected deeper into the dermis.

3. **Belotero Intense** – Higher concentration of hyaluronic acid (25.5mg/ml). The higher concentration is ideal for deeper injection for deep lines such as naso-labial folds, marionette lines, cheeks or increased volume to other areas of the face.

(+) – Any Belotero that has the addition of lidocaine has a '+' sign after the name.

Elevess

Elevess is a hyaluronic acid filler that was FDA approved in 2006 and was the first hyaluronic acid filler to come mixed with lidocaine. This filler has a higher degree of cross-linking and concentration. Its properties make it well suited for deeper injection into the naso-labial fold and marionette line areas.

Comparisons

I have posted many comparisons on my website as well as through different social media platforms and blogs. Nothing seems to interest people as much as hearing how one product may or may not be better than another.

Radiesse vs. Juvederm Voluma

Back in 2006, Radiesse was FDA approved for *subdermal implantation for correction of moderate to severe facial wrinkles and folds (such as nasolabial folds)*. I have been very happy with the results achieved with this product. Radiesse works well for naso-labial folds as well as off-label areas such as marionette lines and cheek augmentation.

Juvederm Voluma was approved in October of 2013 *for deep injection for cheek augmentation to correct age-related volume deficit in the mid-face in adults over the age of 21.* How does Radiesse's 'off label' use for cheek augmentation compare to Juvederm Voluma's FDA approved use?

Unlike Restylane which is injected intra-dermally (into the dermis) for correction of the naso-labial folds, injections for cheek augmentation are placed much deeper. In many cases they are placed right above the cheek bone (the 'periostium'). So the ability of the product to adhere to the periostium and lift the surrounding tissue while augmenting the cheeks really depends to a great extent on its 'lifting' effect. As you recall a higher G-Prime helps 'lift.' Radiesse has a high G-Prime. Radiesse and Juvederm Voluma both want to be recognized for their superior ability to augment the cheek area.

Lifting Effect:

Juvederm Voluma's 'lifting' effect, as discussed is based on its variable molecular sizes and ability to intercollate with and adhere to surrounding tissue.

Radiesse has been used for its lifting effect for many years. It is composed of hydroxylapatite (a component of bone and cartilage) and is the heaviest of all dermal fillers. It too gives a strong lifting effect. It appears as though both of these fillers have this lifting effect, as to which lifts *more*, it is too close to call.

Bottom line is if you are looking for cheek augmentation, your injector should be using Radiesse, Juvederm Voluma or Restylane Lyft. They all lift and work beautifully.

How Long They Last:

Juvederm Voluma's company (Allergan) states it lasts "up to 2 years." I feel this designation is a valid one. I tend to tell people to expect 18 month duration. However, if more is injected at a single setting (i.e. 2 + syringes to a given area), 2 years is certainly possible. Radiesse typically lasts 12-18 months. I have seen Radiesse last 18 months quite frequently.

Personally I prefer a range vs. an "up to" designation. My experience is that in terms of filler duration, Juvederm Voluma has a slight edge. There are other factors to consider. It depends on how quickly the product is broken down, activity level, skill of the injector and amount injected. In the study where Juvederm Voluma was shown to last up to 2 years, large volumes were injected. In defense of Allergan it is important to realize they are not giving a 2 year guarantee, they are saying it is *possible*. Radiesse does not make that claim and perhaps has a more easily understood 'range.'

Cost:

The average cost of Radiesse is approximately $600 to $800 and comes in a 1.5ml syringe.

The cost of Juvederm Voluma XC is $750-1000+ and comes in a 2.0 ml syringe.

Cost varies incredibly depending on where you live. If your doctor is in New York City, expect the high end. I have seen Radiesse priced as low as $500 and Voluma as high as $1200. Fact is, even though Voluma costs more, you *get* more.

Advantages:

Advantage Voluma – Being composed of hyaluronic acid does allow for the use of *hyaluronidase* to dissolve the filler if needed. This has not been a common concern in my medical aesthetic office. It is worth mentioning as an advantage for Voluma. Hence, Voluma has the ability to be reversed to some level if there is a problem or poor result. Radiesse does not have the ability to be dissolved.

Slight advantage Voluma – Juvederm Voluma comes pre-mixed with Lidocaine which improves patient comfort during injection. Radiesse would have to be mixed with lidocaine by an injector familiar with this technique.

Advantage Radiesse – Radiesse, due to its composition, indeed stimulates collagen, whereas Juvederm Voluma does not. However, as is the case with all hyaluronic fillers, Juvederm Voluma will indeed draw water toward itself more so than Radiesse.

Conclusions:

Patients are fortunate to have options and I agree that Voluma's Vycross technology is brilliant. It clearly has broken some new ground as the only dermal filler FDA approved for cheek augmentation. Radiesse is a fantastic option since it lifts well, is of similar cost and stimulates collagen production. I would give a slight edge to Voluma in this head to head comparison. However, both products are excellent choices for marionette lines, nasolabial folds and cheek augmentation.

Belotero vs. Restylane

As discussed, attributes of a dermal filler including cross-linking, particle size, concentration, G-prime and Tyndall effect will determine how and where the dermal filler placement will best help the person being injected. In terms of dermal filler concentrations:

- Belotero Balance – 22.5mg/ml (1.0ml syringe)
- Juvederm Ultra – 24.0mg/ml (0.8ml syringe)
- Restylane – 20mg/ml (1.0ml syringe)
- Restylane Lyft - 20 mg/ml (1.0ml syringe)

As you can see, Restylane has a lower concentration (as well as lower molecular size) which makes it ideal for lips, fine lines and tear troughs. Restylane Lyft, despite the same concentration, has more cross-linking and a larger molecular size which makes it more aptly suited to fill areas which require a larger volume to be filled (cheeks, naso-labial folds, marionette lines). While concentration is important, it is not the only factor to consider.

Belotero, the Tyndall Effect and G-Prime

Belotero has a low G-Prime with variable cross-linking. This makes it far less likely to cause the Tyndall effect when injected superficially. This is an advantage based on science. However, it is important to note that the presence or absence of a Tyndall effect is highly injector dependent and any filler that is placed very superficially may result in this effect.

How Long They Last

Belotero claims to last longer than Restylane or Juvederm (up to 12 months). After speaking with other cosmetic surgeons and medical aesthetic physicians, reviewing case reports (as well as my own experience), I will tell you that Belotero, Restylane and Juvederm all last an average of six months, sometimes more, sometimes less. How long a filler lasts is dependent on many factors:

- Amount injected
- Where injected (i.e. lips do not last as long as cheeks, naso-labial folds or tear troughs)
- The experience, expertise and technique of your injector.
- Activity level
- Maintenance of adequate hydration. Remember, hyaluronic acid draws water to itself, so someone who is well hydrated will typically get more life to their filler.

Fine Lines and Wrinkles

Belotero and Restylane are excellent choices for fine lines, wrinkles and tear troughs. I have not had problems with the Tyndall effect when injecting Restylane superficially but am well aware and have seen documented cases that it indeed does occur. My feeling is that these two are quite equivalent. I see no huge benefit of one over the other as far as filling in fine lines and wrinkles or use in the lips. Belotero can correct any area as well as Restylane and vice versa.

Results

The makers of Belotero argue that a lower viscosity, lower G-prime and variable cross-linking equate to quicker results. With the exception of Sculptra, all dermal fillers I have discussed give immediate results. How natural these results may be is highly dependent on the skill of the person performing the injections. Cost differences between Belotero and Restylane are negligible.

The Verdict – No Winner

Belotero and Restylane both are excellent products. They are effective dermal fillers for the treatment of naso-labial folds, marionette lines, lips, lip lines, tear troughs and other fine facial lines. There is less chance for a blue discoloration (Tyndall effect) after superficial injections with Belotero but this effect with Restylane is really quite rare.

Radiesse for the Hands

In June of 2015, Radiesse seriously broke new ground as the first dermal filler in history to be FDA approved for any area other than the face. Its approval was, *'For hand augmentation to correct volume loss in the dorsum (backs) of the hands.'*

The skin of the face and hands has the greatest overall sun exposure on the body. Certainly in medical aesthetics we focus on improvements of the face. We have neurotoxins like Botox and Dysport, a host of dermal fillers and a wide variety of laser treatments available. These along with microdermabrasion, chemical peels and skin care products give us one heck of an arsenal for anti-aging, reversal of sun damage and treatment of chronic skin conditions like acne, melasma and rosacea. Spotted and wrinkled hands can make someone appear older despite a beautiful and youthful facial appearance. Apparently someone at Merz Aesthetics thought addressing aged hands was a fantastic idea and the use of Radiesse seemed to be a very viable option.

Making Hands Look Younger

If someone wants more youthful-appearing hands the first step is intense pulsed light (IPL) treatments to the back of the hands to help clear sun damage (age spots). I have found that over 80% of those with age-related volume loss to the back of their hands, also have sun damage. The next step is to inject Radiesse into the dorsum of the hands to improve the smoothness and contour of the hands.

This procedure to inject Radiesse into the hands can be costly as it is common for each hand to need one 1.5ml syringe of Radiesse which on average is $600-$800/syringe. Thus, this procedure, which should last about a year, is going to run at minimum $1,200 and likely hundreds more.

I think this is a great procedure. If you couple it with some IPL treatments beforehand, you are definitely going to have much younger looking hands. However, injection into the hands brings a few potential complications that aren't necessarily present in the face. Hence, like I have said many times before; make sure your injector is experienced and well trained with this type of injection.

Potential Problems

The backs of the hands have veins and tendons. Injection into a tendon can weaken it and potentially cause tendon rupture. Injection into a vein can cause emboli where the product travels outside the hands. Nearly half of people (48%) notice subtle changes in their ability to use their hands and about 12% notice nodules or bumps which may last for months. Personally, I would be OK with IPL, but since I am writing, typing or doing injections so much I suspect I wouldn't want the potential aggravation of issues with my hands.

Treating the hands to make them appear more youthful may not be for everyone. While I am all for the time and money spent by women to beautify their nails, on occasion spending some of that money to beautify the hands as well can make a very big difference.

The Vampire Facelift

The American Society of Plastic Surgeons data in 2015 revealed continued growth in surgical and medical aesthetic procedures. Of the nearly 16 million procedures performed, 88% of those were non-surgical with Botox and dermal fillers leading the list. One of these non-surgical procedures receiving a great deal of press is the so-called **Vampire Facelift**. The term 'Vampire Facelift' specifically refers to a procedure whereby both a hyaluronic acid filler as well as platelet rich plasma (PRP) are injected into the face for increased volume and to fill-in areas of deficit (wrinkles). However, many similar procedures including the injection of PRP alone or PRP as SELPHYL® are also referred to by both practitioners and patients as a 'Vampire Facelift.' Before further description I would like to take a closer look at its name.

Vampire

With movies and television series such as "Twilight" and "American Horror Story" the vampire scene is very hip and trendy. No…you don't need to be a vampire or visit one to get a vampire facelift.

However describing the vampire facelift you just had is certainly more sexy and edgy than your friend who received "a syringe of Restylane." The fact that Kim Kardashian showed the world her vampire facelift didn't hurt the buzz about it either.

Facelift

A facelift is when there is surgical repositioning of tissues of the face. Plastic or cosmetic surgeons performing facelifts use scalpels to make incisions and sew tissue into place using sutures. Restylane is an injection. A Vampire Facelift is an injection **not** a facelift. I am certain despite my displeasure with the name of this treatment it will continue to be called a 'Vampire Facelift.'

Again a "true" Vampire Facelift involves the injection of both platelet rich plasma as well as a hyaluronic acid dermal filler such as Juvederm.

Platelet Rich Plasma (PRP)

Platelet rich plasma (PRP) was first developed in the 1970s. It has been used since 2006 in cosmetic medicine for anti-aging and facial rejuvenation. Platelets are known best for their ability to clot blood. However, platelets also release growth factors and cytokines. These growth factors increase the proliferation of cells that repair the skin. They increase collagen production and aid tissue regeneration. Cytokines are cells that improve the communication between cells while helping to move reparative cells to these areas.

PRP is obtained by drawing blood from the patient. This blood is then put into a vial which is centrifuged. This separates the white and red blood cell components from the remaining serum and platelets which, in effect, is PRP. This can be applied to the face during microneedling procedures or injected into areas of the face. From 9 ccs of blood drawn, one typically can get 4-5 ccs of PRP.

SELPHYL® and Platelet Rich Fibrin Matrix

This system incorporates another step into the process whereby calcium chloride turns the liquid platelet rich plasma (PRP) into a gel-like matrix. It accomplishes this through the conversion of fibrinogen to fibrin during an "activation" step. This PRP now becomes what is known as Platelet Rich Fibrin Matrix (PRFM). This is then injected into certain areas of the face.

Occasionally patients are squeamish about getting their blood drawn. Injecting the patient's own serum/blood would appear to be very natural and without side effects. However, you are injecting blood products into a place where it is not typically present in the body. Due to this fact, some may experience burning and itching of the area after the PRP, Selphyl or any other 'vampire' injection.

The Vampire Facelift does not show immediate results. The full effect typically occurs by week three. With dermal fillers, the results are immediate. Dermal fillers have been studied extensively and are well trusted to give predictable results. Such is not the case with the Vampire Facelift, PRP or Selphyl injections. Studies backing up the results of the Vampire Facelift are sparse in comparison to that seen with dermal fillers.

While I am not a fan of the term "Vampire Facelift," it is certainly a viable option in terms of another dermal filler approach. I am very familiar and certainly a fan of the use of PRP with microneedling. If I was given a choice of getting a Vampire Facelift or 2ccs of Juvederm Voluma, I would choose that latter.

Comforts and Cautions

I have used many approaches to ensure patient comfort while performing dermal filler injections. For a period of time I used dental blocks, similar to what you may have at the dentist office. This was problematic for patients. The injection itself was very uncomfortable and people remained numb for hours after leaving the office.

I have found that topical anesthesia works best. It is applied directly onto the skin for about 20-30 minutes before the procedure. During this time it absorbs into the skin causing a very effective local anesthesia. It is fully cleaned off before the procedure but the skin remains numb for about 30-45 minutes.

Lidocaine with epinephrine is one option. It does an excellent job of numbing the area plus the epinephrine constricts small arteries resulting in less bleeding and/or bruising.

Another topical anesthetic is "BLT Cream." This is also known as 'Triple Numbing Cream.' It is called BLT because it contains 20% Benzocaine, 6% Lidocaine and 4% Tetracaine. This combination has been shown to be effective since benzocaine and tetracaine have a very rapid onset of action while lidocaine has a more medium to long duration of action.

Also, most hyaluronic fillers come with a standard preparation and one pre-mixed with lidocaine (i.e. Restylane-L). This does not negate pain when the needle penetrates the skin. That is purpose of the *topical anesthetic*. Dermal fillers with lidocaine have the benefit of patient comfort during the actual filler injection and after, when the injector is smoothening out the area. A good injector should always do this.

Despite the ease and comfort most experience with the use of topical anesthetics, some individuals prefer to feel no pain whatsoever and prefer a dental block. Speak with your injector about your pain tolerance and to discuss what options they are able to provide.

Dermal fillers should not be injected in pregnant or nursing patients, those taking aspirin or blood thinners or with a history of bruising easily. People should not take aspirin, Aleve (naproxen), Advil (ibuprofen), vitamin E or St. John's Wort *for one week before to 2-3 days after* the procedure. Tylenol (acetaminophen) is OK. I have used arnica tablets frequently to help reduce the likelihood of bruising. Eating some large pieces of pineapple frankly has the same effect as arnica. If people have cold sores, I prefer they are treated and resolved before I inject. Neither topical anesthetics nor dermal fillers should be injected if skin infection is present.

Since the injector is putting a needle through the skin there is the risk of infection, bleeding, bruising, swelling and pain. Typically bruising and swelling subside in 3-7 days. Infections are exceedingly rare.

The most important factor to prevent complications and to help insure a beautiful result is the experience and track record of your injector. Do your homework. Ask questions.

- How long have you been injecting?

- What products are you most comfortable injecting?

- How do you handle requests for touch ups?

- What fillers do you recommend for different areas of the face?

A good injector should be able to thoroughly answer these questions and more.

Chapter Eight

Anti-Aging Laser (and other) Treatments

There are many ways indeed to treat one's face in an attempt to restore or accentuate beauty. Entire volumes have been written on the subject of cosmetic laser treatments. There have been dramatic improvements over the past ten years in the ability of lasers to rejuvenate the skin. Lasers can be used to tighten the skin, reduce the presence of sun damage, remove unwanted hair and treat acne and other chronic skin conditions. With the exception of laser hair removal, when I discuss cosmetic laser treatments with a patient, I always interject the need for a comprehensive approach.

For instance, if someone would like Intense Pulsed Light treatments to clear away unwanted pigment, I will also discuss the use of sunblock as well as other treatments that will keep the skin well hydrated following the procedure.

If a patient begins body contouring or cellulite reduction treatments, I incorporate a new diet and exercise plan for them. In fact, simply doing repeated body contouring procedures without an accompanying diet plan is really doing a disservice to the patient.

Back when I was in primary care, it was of paramount importance to discuss diet and exercise as part of the treatment for diabetes. In fact, health maintenance was discussed during any type of visit. In today's fast paced primary care environment, it is frequently missed or if mentioned it's with a casual "keep an eye on your weight" comment. Hence, it is no surprise that the incidence of obesity and diabetes continues to rise every year in the US.

Point is, the vast majority of laser procedures are simply 'helpers.' They are not stand alone treatments. If a person is relying solely on laser procedures to attain a youthful result, they are apt to be quite disappointed.

Intense Pulsed Light (IPL)

IPL was first introduced in 1995. It was used to treat telangectasias (dilated capillaries near the surface of the skin commonly called 'spider veins'). In 1996 IPL was used in Germany to treat individuals with Port Wine Stain (a birthmark caused by dilated blood vessels giving the skin a red-purple discoloration). Soon thereafter it was shown to be effective at removing unwanted hair.

Knowing the history of IPL shows how medicine progresses. 20 years ago this device was shown to be effective vs. red discolorations. Now, IPL is a versatile and capable means for treatment of a multitude of skin concerns which include:

1. Brown pigmented lesions – age spots, freckles and erythromelanosis (poikiloderma)
2. Red discolorations – spider veins, rosacea, broken capillaries, telangectasias
3. Hair removal
4. Pre-cancerous lesions – actinic keratosis, Bowen's disease
5. Photorejuvination/Anti-Aging – IPL stimulates fibroblasts in the dermis to increase production of collagen and elastin. IPL

therefore will give some anti-aging advantage in the wavelengths used for treatment of red and/or brown discolorations.

6. In some cases will improve acne

How Does IPL Work?

Intense Pulsed Light (IPL) devices produce high energy light sources via a flash-lamp. These lamps produce a *high energy broad wavelength output*; typically between 500-1200 nanometers. This light energy is targeted to specific areas of the skin. Since these devices are placed directly upon the skin, they are cooled to help protect it.

The light energy is transferred to target cells which are skin cells with color (so-called 'chromophores'). The light energy is converted to heat energy which damages and disrupts the architecture of the targeted cell. IPL uses many wavelengths (colors) in each pulse of light along with a filter that refines the light output.

Targets:

With hair removal, the laser is attaining a deeper penetration into the dermis where the pigment of the hair follicle lies. This is the area we want to disrupt to cause the hair to literally fall out. With red discolorations the chromophore we are going after is hemoglobin. With brown discolorations we are targeting melanin.

Advice before the Procedure:

1. You should avoid the sun for at least two weeks before the procedure or be wearing SPF 50 sunblock. IPL should not be used on those with skin redness as it increases the likelihood that the laser will be irritating to (or even burn) the skin surface.
2. Bruising is a rare side effect of IPL and avoidance of aspirin, Advil and Aleve for a week prior will further reduce the likelihood of this happening.
3. IPL should not be performed during pregnancy.

What to Expect During an IPL Treatment:

1. A topical anesthetic may be applied for 20-30 minutes. This is removed, followed by the application of a cool gel to the area to be treated. This gel is similar to that used when an expectant mother has an ultrasound. This allows the laser to have full contact with the area of skin being treated.
2. Treatments last from 15-60 minutes depending on the size of the area treated.
3. You will wear protective glasses or eye pads.
4. As the pulses of light are being sent from the laser into your skin, you will feel a sensation similar to a rubber band snapping or slight stinging.
5. When the treatment is completed, the gel will be removed with a cool cloth and the attendant should apply a moisturizer with sun block.
6. Occasionally, if there is some warmth or discomfort of the skin following the treatment a cool compress may be applied.

What to Expect After the Procedure:

1. If you were treated for brown discolorations such as age spots or freckles, the spots actually will look darker for 5-7 days. Next the disrupted cells containing melanin move up to the skin surface and literally 'flake off' as they are ultimately cleared.
2. For treatment of red areas such as broken capillaries or telangectasias, the skin may actually appear red for 3-5 days and then will begin to clear. The hemoglobin is broken down resorbed primarily through the blood stream.
3. There is no need to restrict activity in any way following and IPL or the use of makeup.
4. One should wear a minimum of SPF 20 as the skin remains somewhat more prone to sunburn immediately after the procedure.

The Cost of an IPL Treatment:

One of the main reasons IPL can be expensive is that typically it takes several treatments to attain optimal results. I tell patients 3-5 treatments for brown and red discolorations or laser hair removal. If a man needs laser hair removal to his entire back, it is going to take more treatments and will be more expensive than a woman who wants a spot treatment to pesky chin hairs that keep recurring.

For example, a full face IPL treatment will typically cost about $300-$500. These treatments are spaced one month apart. Therefore a full face treatment will typically run an average of $1000-$2000. As is the case with any medical aesthetic treatment, you are going to pay more depending on the zip code of where you are receiving these treatments. More expensive doesn't necessarily equate to a better treatment. Larger cities such as Chicago, Los Angeles and New York City tend to be more expensive as a general rule.

Be Clear

Whether your goal is photorejuvenation, brown spots, red discolorations or hair removal make certain you clearly explain to the laser specialist exactly what your goals of these treatments are. Further, make sure your laser technician is well versed in treating the areas of concern you have.

If the laser treatments seem extremely cheap, the specialist can't explain the details of the procedure or does not have any evidence of certification for the use of the laser, please leave. You don't have to look far to see some very bad outcomes (burns) caused by those using a laser without the proper training.

The Laser I Use Most

IPL is one of my favorite laser procedures and I am not alone. IPL has shown a 44% increase in popularity in the past 5 years. IPL addresses so many different dermatologic concerns in an effective and relatively painless manner with little or no downtime. The beauty of having IPL for treatment of red or brown discolorations is that you get a little anti-aging boost as the heat energy from the laser stimulates fibroblasts to make more collagen and elastin. The result is tighter skin with fewer brown or red discolorations.

Laser Hair Removal

Laser hair removal may not be the most exciting or glamorous procedure in medical aesthetics, but it certainly is popular. There were 828,000 laser hair removal treatments performed in 2014 making it the third most commonly sought after treatment. Hair is an interesting part of the skin. Women and men both spend a great deal of time, money and energy on issues related to their hair. Having a gorgeous head of hair is glamorous. Having the right hair in the right places can be something striking, sexy and beautiful and can even make a statement about who you are.

A European study showed that the average woman spends $650 a year or about $40,000 during her adult life on hair care products and treatments. Men spend far less on hair styling. As a group, men dish out over a billion dollars a year in an attempt to improve hair loss. The most expensive treatment is a hair transplant, followed by topical treatments such as Rogaine, medications such as Propecia, vitamin supplements and toupees/hairpieces. The use of peptides and microneedling is also showing early promise in the treatment of hair loss in men (and women).

Laser Hair Removal is Actually Quite Interesting

Laser hair removal was performed experimentally for about 20 years before it became a mainstream procedure in the mid-1990s. Through the years, I have used several different lasers for hair removal including the Lumenis Lightsheer and Alma Soprano. The cooled laser head certainly helps with patient comfort. Women most commonly come in for removal of hair from the lip, chin, underarms and bikini area and less commonly for the arms, legs and breasts. Men (frequently after a push from their significant other) come in for hair removal of back, shoulder, upper arm and chest hair. Some women love hairy chests, some love beards, some love both, some hate both. Women seem to come in for laser hair removal on their own accord while men are frequently coerced.

Understanding Laser Hair Removal:

The truth is that laser hair removal should really be described as *permanent hair reduction.* In many (but not all) cases it removes all the hair in the area treated – permanently. Success requires a skilled laser technician and multiple treatments. When attempting to destroy a hair follicle the goal is to disrupt the germ cells residing on the surface of the hair shaft. This is accomplished by the laser's light energy being absorbed by melanin and generating heat. This process results in destruction of the germ cells and the hair ultimately falling out.

The hairs which are most damaged by this process are the ones *in the growth stage.* There are several stages hair follicles pass through. These include the Anagen (growth), Catagen (transition), and Telogen (resting) phases. Hair cells in the Anagen (growth) stage have active germ cells and a high melanin content, hence the laser hits them very well …but only them. Thus, multiple treatments are needed to strike every hair in its Anagen phase.

Melanin is highest in the bulb of the hair and is a *chromophore* (what gives a substance its color). In the case of laser hair removal the chromophore of the hair is melanin, specifically *Eumelanin.* There are two types of melanin in regard to laser hair removal:

1. Eumelanin – gives hair a black or brown color
2. Pheomelanin – gives hair a blonde or red color.

Because the actual photons of light from the laser are chasing eumelanin, it stands to reason that black or brown hair, with the highest eumelanin content, respond best to laser hair removal treatments. The most ideal situation is someone who is light skinned with dark coarse hair. The light energy penetrates the surface of the skin and targets the eumelanin in the hair follicle. Once the follicle is hit by the laser and disrupted in the Anagen phase, the hair follicle falls out and no further hair can grow from that area. Multiple sessions are needed, essentially to get each and every hair follicle when it is at an Anagen phase, and to hit any missed in earlier treatments. It is best to space the treatments apart by about 3-5 weeks and it is not uncommon to need five or more treatments depending on the area. It is important to reiterate that the experience of the laser technician is important to help assure the area treated is covered thoroughly, systematically and safely.

Better Candidates:

Light skin with dark hair is the ideal situation. Lasers do not work as well with lighter colored hair, blonde hair, red hair (pheomelanin) or fine hair. Since the laser targets melanin, it is also difficult to perform laser hair removal on patients with darker skin types. Lasers are not that smart. They cannot tell the difference between melanin in the hair follicle and that in the skin.

The Fitzpatrick Classification describes six skin types. Laser hair removal can be performed very well, for the most part, on skin types I, II, III & IV. In some cases an Nd:Yag laser with a cooling tip may be helpful in treating darker (V, VI) skin types when used by an experienced practitioner. The use of steroid cream (anti-inflammatory) has also shown to help with laser hair removal with Fitzpatrick types V and VI. With these darker skin types the hair removal tends to be less complete and more side effects are reported.

The Fitzpatrick Scale		
Fitzpatrick	**Characteristics**	**Skin type**
Type I	Never tans, always burns	Extremely fair skin
Type II	Occasionally tans, usually burns	Fair skin
Type III	Tans average, sometimes burns	Medium skin
Type IV	Usually tans, rarely burns	Olive skin
Type V	Mostly tans, almost never burns	Dark brown skin
Type VI	Never burns	Black skin

Prior to Treatment:

1. Discuss your treatment with the doctor, nurse or aesthetician who is about to perform this procedure and ask to see their certification to operate the machine they will be using. This is standard and nobody should be surprised by this request. Much like what I discussed in regard to IPL techs, a poorly trained

laser operator for laser hair removal can cause big problems, including burns.

2. Do not pluck, wax or dye the hair you wish to be treated and do not sun tan for at least one month prior to any treatment.

After Treatment:

1. Hairs should be allowed to fall out and should not be pulled on as this can cause increased skin irritation and possibly infection.

2. Patients should use SPF 20+ vs. UVA/UVB rays to sun exposed areas that have been treated.

Possible Side Effects:

1. Common side effects include pink skin, itching and minimal swelling.

2. Changes in pigmentation can occur in rare cases (*hypo*pigmentation or *hyper*pigmentation).

3. Similar to IPL, the procedure itself may feel like a rubber band snapping or stinging sensation which can be lessened by the use of anesthetic creams such as BLT. Of note, a laser technician should never cover a very large area (i.e. back/chest) with strong numbing creams due to potentially serious cardiac side effects which can occur.

Alternatives:

Laser hair removal is a very mainstream procedure. However, people still rely on other measures such as tweezing, waxing, bleaching, electrolysis and topical creams. Waxing is a very common treatment. It can be quite painful and result in skin tears. It also really doesn't work well on shorter hairs.

Electrolysis is a painful and tedious means of removing hair follicles individually. There are many electrolysis practitioners that are very good at what they do and swear by this procedure. While I have never used electrolysis as part of my practice, there is a population that does very well with it. The benefit of electrolysis is that each individual hair is removed regardless of what stage (anagen, catagen, telogen) the hair follicle is in.

Vaniqua (ornithine decarboxylase) is a topical cream that prevents hair growth. The active ingredient (eflornithine hydrochloride) accomplishes this chemically. Data submitted to the FDA showed that about 58% of women using the cream on facial hair had improvement. This may not be a bad option for those who do not want a laser hair removal procedure. However, it is not going to clear hair follicles as well as a laser.

While I primarily treat people's faces, laser hair removal is a big part of what clients want to enhance their beauty. Talk with the professional who is performing your laser treatment about your expectations and to get an idea how many treatments may be needed to give optimal results. As laser technologies continue to improve, it will become increasingly possible to safely and effectively treat darker skin types and lighter hair colors.

Fraxel

The Fraxel Laser is a type of laser which accomplishes something commonly described as *laser skin resurfacing*. This type of laser literally makes thousands of tiny holes (or columns) through the epidermis into the dermis. The skin areas between the holes are unaffected. This approach allows the skin to heal more quickly than if the entire surface of the skin was treated. Through this type of laser treatment, the skin's natural healing process results in the growth of a new 'surface' to the top layer of the skin (epidermis).

Since the laser extends into the dermis it results in the stimulation of fibroblasts which produce more collagen and elastin. The end result is a fresh skin surface and a boost of the supporting architecture of collagen and elastin in the dermis. I also had the opportunity to use a Pixel laser (Alma) which is another version of the Fraxel laser. Fraxel is beneficial over traditional CO2 laser procedures in that the laser penetrates more deeply into the skin layers while leaving the majority of the skin surface intact. Some Fraxel lasers (known as 'dual wavelength') offer the additional benefit of a secondary wavelength which targets unwanted pigment much as an IPL laser treatment does.

Fraxel Benefits:

1. Improvement of fine lines and wrinkles
2. Improvement of acne or other scars
3. Reduction of pigmented areas (age spots, freckles or sun spots)
4. Clearance of pre-cancerous skin conditions (actinic keratosis)

Before the Procedure:

The primary advice I give is to avoid sun exposure for several weeks before treatment. If the skin is red and inflamed prior to treatment, there will be an increased potential for skin irritation or even infection. While not a universal practice, some practitioners prescribe an anti-viral (to avoid cold sores) and/or antibiotics for 3-5 days after treatment. Pregnant patients or those taking Accutane should not have Fraxel treatments. Patients with very dark skin types (Fitzpatrick V-VI) may undergo Fraxel with extreme caution in the hands of an experienced laser operator. Those who are prone to form scars (keloids) should not undergo Fraxel.

The Procedure:

Thorough cleansing of the skin is of paramount important with this and any other medical aesthetic procedure. A topical anesthetic should be applied to the area to be treated. This anesthetic should be left on for a minimum of 20-30 minutes before commencing.

The hand piece of the laser will be passed over the face. This should be done in a systematic fashion. If there are areas of particular concern, the laser may be passed over these areas more than once. There is a pattern to this. Remember, we want to have the laser go over areas of the face once, so if the laser operator is not systematic in their approach, some areas may be covered too much while others not covered enough. The laser has a cooling device to blow cold air to cool the skin as it is treated. During the procedure your skin may feel hot at times or have a 'prickling' or 'stinging' sensation. There is occasionally some pinpoint bleeding but this is not common. While the procedure is typically done to the face, other areas such as neck, chest, arms, hands or anywhere scars are present may be treated.

After Treatment:

The skin should be cleansed again after the procedure and cooling of the skin with soft ice packs is very helpful. The most common side effects are redness and swelling, which will slowly subside over the course of 5-7 days. Other symptoms include itching, dryness or a bronzed skin appearance. Peeling and flaking of the skin is quite common as the epidermis is making an entirely new surface (hence the name laser *resurfacing)*. After the procedure it is very important to keep your skin well moisturized. Fraxel does an amazing job of skin rejuvenation. However, it does make the skin very dry in the process. Products with hyaluronic acid, glycerin or petroleum are very helpful after the procedure to keep the skin well hydrated. Sun exposure should be avoided and once the skin begins to heal, SPF 30+ vs. UVA/UVB rays may be applied as well.

Results:

Ideally one will see results following one treatment however multiple treatments will give more marked results. These are typically spaced apart by at least 4 weeks. I recommend three treatments, spaced one month apart. As the skin continues to heal and fibroblasts continue to form more collagen and elastin, results continue for many months following a series of treatments. These treatments are best maintained by keeping the skin moisturized daily and avoiding UVA/UVB rays.

A Fraxel laser can give amazing results when used by a well trained and experienced laser operator. Unlike IPL or laser hair removal where multiple treatments are typically recommended at the outset, I take a 'one Fraxel at a time' approach with most patients. Nothing says you need to have a series of three or more treatments. Many people are quite satisfied with one treatment. There is down time with these treatments as the skin will commonly be red and irritated with skin flaking for 5-7 days or more.

Microneedling – An Alternative to Fraxel

Microneedling is a procedure gaining incredible momentum in the medical aesthetic world. New or updated devices are being released at a steady pace, each claiming to be superior to all others on the market. Environ™, led by plastic surgeon Des Fernandez, MD, introduced their microneedling roller as far back as 1996 for treatment of fine lines around the mouth. So why is microneedling increasing in popularity? I see six main reasons.

1. It is an effective means of treating a wide array of common skin concerns.
2. It is less expensive than laser skin resurfacing. We all know laser treatments are expensive; because lasers are *very expensive*. The cost for buying or leasing a laser will rival most home mortgages. Don't get me wrong, I am a fan of cosmetic laser treatments but I am also a realist. Most people will choose to get tangible results for less money when possible.
3. There is far less downtime with microneedling vs. laser skin resurfacing.
4. Unlike chemical peels, microneedling can be used on any skin type.
5. Studies have shown microneedling to be a simple and inexpensive method for the treatment of facial scars.
6. Microneedling creates hundreds of micro-channels allowing for enhanced penetration of skin care products deep into the dermis.

How Microneedling Works

Microneedling is a procedure whereby thousands of tiny holes are punctured in the skin. It is 'controlled skin injury.' These holes or 'micro-wounds' trigger the body to fill in these holes by producing new collagen and elastin in the dermis along with new capillaries. The new blood flow and collagen production results in improvement of scars and rejuvenation of the skin. The texture, firmness and hydration of the skin are improved. Microneedling is also referred to as collagen induction therapy (CIT) which is a very accurate description of what is happening. The depth of the needle penetration dictates the level of injury to the skin and the potential results to be achieved. Microneedling literally helps the skin help itself.

Microneedling – Broken Down into Steps:

1. **Inflammation** (day 1-3)

   The initial injury to the skin causes platelets to respond along with growth factors, other healing cells and new capillaries. Other cells come to the area to remove debris. Cells of the upper skin layer (epidermis) divide and new fibroblasts are stimulated in the dermal layer.

2. **Proliferation** (day 4-6)

   The new vibrant cells of the epidermis and fibroblasts of the dermis continue to multiply and proliferate.

3. **Maturation** (day 7-28)

   Fibroblasts form collagen and elastin in the dermis giving more tightness and tone to the skin while the cells of the epidermis flourish giving a smoother and more uniform surface.

4. **From Day 28 +**

   A new healthy skin surface is present while the collagen and elastin of the dermis continue to 'tighten' further improving the firmness of the skin.

Types of Devices

1. **Hand Held Rollers**

These devices have been around for a very long time. Along with the growth of microneedling in the medical spa world has come a host of 'home based' microneedling rollers. These are commonly sold with skin care product lines. These do not achieve the needle depth of more advanced electrical systems but are indeed a helpful and economical approach. Products can be used with mechanical rollers allowing them to penetrate more deeply into the skin.

2. Battery Powered / Electrical Devices

These devices are able to penetrate the skin more deeply. Also of note, the needle penetration with these devices is more *vertical.* The holes made with dermal rollers have a tendency to cause more than the necessary damage to the skin surface as a certain percentage of the needles will not penetrate the skin in an exact-vertical manner (i.e. on a slight angle). The electrical devices are typically reserved for use in a medical setting under the care of an aesthetician, nurse or doctor. MicroPen, SkinPen II™, Collagen P.I.N.™, and Rejuvapen® are some of the well-known devices used in medical spas and dermatology/cosmetic surgery practices. They have between 9 and 12 needles, smooth or beveled tips and the ability to change the needle depth from 0.25-3.0 mm. Devices allow for the infusion of different products into the skin during the treatment.

3. Product-Infusing Devices

Aquagold™ Plus is a system that allows for the delivery of cosmeceuticals, plasma rich plasma, antioxidants, retinol, growth factors, hydroquinone, hyaluronic acid, even dilute neurotoxins *during* the microneedling procedure.

However, it should be noted that these products can also be 'infused' into the skin during a microneedling procedure using a standard electrical or battery powered device (i.e. Micropen). For instance, platelet rich plasma (PRP) drawn from the patient can be applied to the skin during the procedure. The product enters the deeper layers of the skin along with the penetration of the needles. Microneedling is an excellent means of product infusion into both the epidermal and dermal layers. For this and many of the aforementioned reasons, microneedling has become very popular. It truly brings amazing anti-aging results. .

What to Expect at a Microneedling Appointment

1. Your face should be cleansed well and numbing (lidocaine/BLT) cream should be applied.
2. The procedure takes anywhere from 10-60 minutes depending on the area of skin being treated.

3. It is relatively painless. Depending on how deep the needles penetrate, in some cases there will be some minor bleeding of the skin.
4. Your face should then be cleansed and gentle moisturizers or serums and sun block may be applied.
5. In the first 48 -72 hours your skin will be red and warm, much like a sun burn. People should avoid strenuous activity and stay out of the sun. Medications such as hydrocortisone 1% can be used to relieve itching and irritation that may be present.
6. After that time your skin should begin to calm down as it begins to heal.

Cautions

1. While your skin is healing, sun exposure should be limited for at least 2 weeks (or use SPF 50).
2. Avoid use of Aspirin or NSAIDS (Advil/Aleve) for 3 days prior to 2 weeks after procedure.
3. Avoid use of Retinol (Vitamin A) creams or serums for 1 week.
4. Skin infections should be fully resolved for 1 week prior to treatment.
5. Microneedling should not be done until 3-4 weeks after Botox, Dysport or dermal filler treatments.
6. Not all needles are the same, and the treatment can be technique dependent. For example, overly aggressive needling may cause scarring and hyperpigmentation in certain skin types.

Conditions Microneedling Treats:

- Fine lines and wrinkles
- Mild to moderate acne scarring, or other scars
- Loose skin (the face, neck, décolleté area)
- Uneven skin texture or large pore size
- Stretch marks

- Melasma / hyperpigmentation

We Have Seen this Before

In medical aesthetics we have seen other types of skin damage resulting in improved skin appearance. Chemical peels, for instance, penetrate through skin layers in an attempt to clear dead cells and stimulate new skin cell and collagen growth. New cells make the skin more vibrant while new collagen (and elastin) makes the skin more smooth and firm.

The Verdict

Microneedling has clearly come of age. It is less expensive, comes with less down time and is less damaging to the skin than laser resurfacing. It improves skin smoothness, tone, elasticity, texture and can also remove unwanted pigment. Unlike chemical peels, it can be performed on all skin types. Mastering proper techniques is important but can be easily learned by those wanting to perform these procedures. Make sure your doctor, nurse or aesthetician is well trained on the use of the device and you are sure to see results with this procedure.

Treating the Double Chin

A 2014 study of the American Society of Dermatologic Surgery showed 65% of adults surveyed said they were unhappy with under-the-chin fullness. Three factors contribute to the double chin. These include genetics, age and weight changes. The fullness is not sudden. It comes on very subtly and becomes more noticeable and problematic through the years. While one may be very physically fit, under-the-chin fullness may persist. Some facial fullness is healthy as not all fat is necessarily bad. Facial fat contains stem cells which are essential for cell renewal and collagen synthesis. While I am a proponent of diet and exercise, in many cases despite a healthy lifestyle, a double chin may persist.

Kybella

Kybella is manufactured by Kythera Biopharmaceuticals and is FDA approved for treating the fat underneath the chin (also known as submental fat). By definition, Kybella is a cytolytic drug. This is defined as *"a drug that causes the dissolution or destruction of a cell."* Kybella is composed of deoxycholic acid which is an exact match to the deoxycholic acid produced by your body to absorb fats.

This treatment therefore allows for the fat dissolving deoxycholic acid to be injected directly into this commonly troublesome fatty area. The approach used is to inject Kybella into multiple areas in an even distribution (grid) into the chin. Kybella injections dissolve the fat cell's membrane, effectively killing the cell. The destroyed fat and cell components are then cleared through the body's lymphatic system.

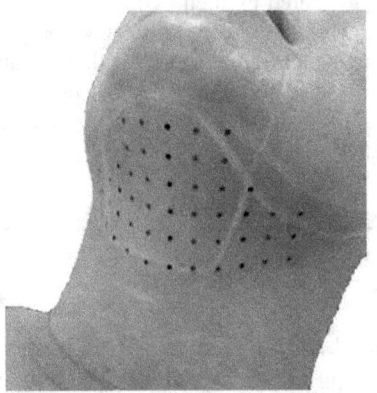

Kybella Chin Grid

When injected correctly into submental fat, the fat cells are destroyed and the chin tightens beautifully. Finding a health care professional well trained and experienced with Kybella is of utmost importance.

Common side effects include injection site reactions (bruising, pain, warmth, swelling, numbness, redness, itching and burning sensations). Less commonly, skin tightness, nerve injury, difficulty swallowing, mouth or throat pain, headache and high blood pressure all have been reported. There are (rare) case reports of nerve damage and resultant facial muscle weakness. An experienced injector is imperative to:

1. Attain a beautiful result
2. Avoid the (rare) serious side effects
3. Reduce the presence *or severity* of (common) post-procedure side effects

Kybella Timeline

1. During the procedure many will experience moderate pain (A '5-7' on a scale of 1-10). Some injectors use a topical anesthetic to ease the discomfort while others use oral pain medication. People typically receive 35-50 injections to the chin area per treatment.
2. Swelling and bruising are the first symptoms people notice beginning shortly after the procedure, peaking at 18-24 hours and resolving by 48 hours. The use of arnica and/or bromelain tablets a day prior to two days after is helpful to reduce bruising. In the first 6-12 hours occasionally people may notice some discomfort with swallowing solid food. Liquids are not typically a problem at any time.
3. At 72-96 hours (3-4 days), people feel the tightening begin as the fat is fully dissolved and cleared through the lymphatic system.
4. By week 3-4 most people will have measurable results in loss of submental (chin) fat. Occasionally there may be mild symptoms of slight tenderness or tingling of the chin area at this time which will indeed continue to resolve in the following weeks.
5. Many experts advise people to have the procedure on a Friday so most of the visible side-effects (redness, swelling, bruising) will be resolved by their return to work Monday.
6. Drinking plenty of fluid is very beneficial to the process as it helps your lymphatic system work more efficiently to clear the dissolved fat cells.

Beyond the Chin

As of this writing, Kybella is undergoing clinical trials to determine its safety and efficacy with the dissolution of abdominal fat. Many doctors are already using Kybella 'off label' to help men achieve 'chiseled abs' without doing hundreds of crunches a day. I have little doubt that in the next 3-5 years (if not sooner) there will be additional indications for Kybella. Currently its FDA approval is for *treatment for adults with moderate-to-severe fat below the chin, known as submental fat.* More indications are coming.

Chin Liposuction

There is a growing list of medical aesthetic procedures to improve the beauty, youth and contour of your face. Kybella may require more than one series of injections. In many cases 3-5 treatments are needed to attain optimal results. At an average of $800-$1200 per treatment the cost of a well contoured chin may add up quickly. A Kybella study of 2,600 patients showed an 80 % satisfaction rate. However, this rate was based on individuals (more than half) *who had 3+ treatments.* My point is that three Kybella treatments may cost you essentially the same as a single chin liposuction treatment.

The average cost of chin liposuction is about $3000 with a range of $2000-$5000. Patient satisfaction rates following chin liposuction are also in the 80-85% range. No two faces are alike and no two chins are alike either. The number of Kybella treatments needed or degree/extent of chin liposuction will depend largely on what your chin is like 'before' and what your desired end result might be. Similarly, a chin that requires 'more work' will certainly be well above the $3000 average chin liposuction price-tag. It is important to consider more than one possible means of treatment when it comes to a double chin.

Another procedure that has been effective in the reduction of submental fat is CoolSculpting.

Coolsculpting

CoolSculpting is quickly becoming one of the most popular noninvasive procedures for double chin reduction. So far, the fat elimination technique has been used over 2 million times. Seven different CoolSculpting attachments are available; each made to treat a different area of the body. The most commonly addressed areas with CoolSculpting include the abdomen, lower back, upper arms, thighs and the double chin.

CoolSculpting's *CoolMini* was approved by the Food and Drug Administration (FDA) as an effective, noninvasive treatment for submental fat. CoolSculpting uses very cold temperatures to kill fat cells. While CoolSculpting can be used in other areas as well, the CoolMini was designed specifically for under the chin, as well as other hard to treat areas.

The very cold temperature from the device effectively numbs the area as the fat in the chin area is targeted. Treatments last approximately 60 minutes. Once these fat cells effectively die, they are cleared through the lymphatic system and metabolized. There are no incisions or needles needed here. However, having this area of your face 'frozen' can be a bit uncomfortable. Each treatment results in a loss of about 20% of the chin fat. This means, again, you will need typically more than one treatment to achieve optimal results.

As always it comes down to knowing about the procedures you are considering along with the results you wish to attain. Be aware of the cost, potential side effects and how satisfied those have been who have had the procedure before. It is my opinion that Kybella, Chin Liposuction as well as Coolsculpting are all viable options to help get rid of that double chin.

LED Light Technology

LED (Light Emitting Diode) light technology encompasses the way certain wavelengths of light and colors can be used to improve the appearance of your skin. It has also been described as photodynamic therapy (or PDT). There is nothing really new about LED therapy. Over 200 years ago a Danish physician (Dr. Neils Finsen) received a Nobel Prize for demonstration of how various wavelengths of light could be used to treat tuberculosis. NASA has used LED technology in space to promote wound healing and tissue growth. LED therapy has been shown in over 40 years of research to be highly beneficial to the skin.

LED Therapy Skin Benefits:

1. Improved circulation in the dermis = improved oxygenation of the skin
2. Increased DNA/RNA synthesis = repair of damaged skin
3. Improved lymphatic activity = clearing of waste and cellular debris
4. Stimulation of fibroblast activity = increased production of collagen and elastin
5. Ability to soothe sun damaged or inflamed skin
6. Improved skin hydration
7. Reduction of pore size
8. Treatment of mild to moderate inflammatory acne and the bacteria associated with it (*P.Acnes*)
9. Skin rejuvenation including improvements of fine lines and wrinkles
10. Improvement of minor scars
11. Improvement of rosacea, melasma, eczema and psoriasis

There are four types of commonly used light therapy which include red, blue, green and amber. Red and blue light treatments are used much more frequently. LED therapy uses wavelengths similar to those used with other traditional lasers but the *delivery of the energy* is far different. LED therapy penetrates the skin and works in a unique way not seen with other laser procedures. However, in many cases similar results can be achieved. LED light therapy is also much less expensive than most laser treatments (i.e. IPL).

Red Light LED Therapy:

Red light therapy (633nm – 830nm) penetrates the human skin to a depth of 8-10mm. This means it gets into the dermis where those fabulous fibroblasts reside. Stimulation of fibroblasts results in an increase in collagen and elastin. Skin layers, because of their high blood and water content absorb this light very well. Red light therapy improves blood flow, which allows for improved oxygenation and nutrient delivery to the cells in the skin. Red light carries strong anti-aging qualities and works on a cellular level.

Potential Benefits of Red Light LED Therapy

1. Increased circulation, oxygenation and nutrient delivery to the skin
2. Increased activity of fibroblasts and collagen/elastin production
3. Improved lymphatic drainage and clearance of wastes from the skin
4. Improved DNA/RNA/ATP synthesis providing energy for healing and skin rejuvenation
5. Reduction in inflammation.
6. Reduction of winkles and fine lines
7. Improvement of Melasma – *The American Journal of Dermatology and Venereology* 2014 demonstrated safe and effective use of red LED (633nm and 830nm) on melasma in skin type VI (darkest skin type). Participants demonstrated improved skin texture, more even tone, reduction of porphyrins, and reduction of fine lines and wrinkles.
8. Improvement of Psoriasis – *Seminars in Cutaneous Medicine and Surgery* (Aug 2014) demonstrated no adverse side effects and a resolution of psoriasis in a patient population that had psoriasis resistant to conventional therapy.

When red LED light is used for facial rejuvenation, treatments are typically performed weekly. More treatments = more results.

Blue Light Therapy

Blue light therapy is of a short wavelength (450-510nm). Blue light is right next to UV light on the electromagnetic spectrum and brings the antibacterial properties of UV light, without the risks associated with UV exposure. Blue light therapy penetrates the skin very superficially (approximately 1 mm). However, it has been shown (and FDA approved) to kill the bacteria associated with some forms of acne (*P. Acnes*). The P. acnes bacteria produce porphyrins as part of its normal metabolism. These porphyrins absorb blue light (and red to a lesser extent) generating reactive oxygen which is toxic to the bacteria.

My opinion is that blue light therapy indeed plays a role with the treatment of acne. The use of blue light therapy combined with the right dietary and topical regimen is a recipe for significant improvement of mild to moderate inflammatory acne. Both blue and red light can be used concomitantly to treat acne. Blue light, as noted though its ability to clear bacteria; red light through its action on a cellular level help reduce inflammation and hasten skin healing.

Blue light, while clearly a means to improve mild to moderate inflammatory acne, is far less affective for cystic acne, blackheads and whiteheads. Clinical trials have shown the need for up to 20 treatments for optimal results (Twice a week for 8 weeks then once a week for four weeks). At $50-100/treatment, this may be an expensive endeavor.

Blue Light Use Number 2

Blue light's second claim to fame is in the treatment of seasonal affective disorder. In 2009 The Journal of Depression and Anxiety showed that blue light treatment was effective in reducing the depression, dysphoria and sleep disturbances seen with this disorder. As far back as 1500 BC, the Greeks were the first to record a suggestion that exposure to light indeed had the potential to "restore health." I have countless patients through the years who have benefited greatly, particularly in the winter months, through the use of blue light therapy.

Green Light Therapy

Green light therapy typically falls in the wavelength range of 515 nm to 520 nm and is most frequently used for skin treatments aimed at anti-aging and removal of unwanted pigment.

In all fairness, the independent research backing up the benefits of green light therapy pale in comparison to what is seen perhaps with red light therapy. Green light therapy can help to fade the appearance of freckles, age spots (or sun spots), brown patches or uneven skin pigment. While green light is indeed an option to consider for clearance of age spots and hyperpigmentation, intense pulsed light (IPL) is far and away more effective.

Amber Light Therapy:

This is also known as yellow or orange light therapy. It has been shown to be beneficial in treatment of skin redness, irritation and small veins (telangectasias). I think of amber light as more of a 'calming' treatment for red, irritated skin. It also helps improved lymphatic drainage and flushes waste from the skin.

LED Therapy vs. Intense Pulsed Light (IPL)

Like the name implies IPL stands for '*Intense* pulsed light.' While LED may employ similar wavelengths to IPL, the delivery of the energy is far different. IPL pulses are delivered at a high energy over a fraction of a second. This means there is certainly a higher chance of a burn as well as pain with IPL treatments. IPL is my preferred treatment for clearance of brown pigment on lighter skin types. LED energy is of a similar wavelength to that seen with IPL however this energy is delivered very slowly over an extended period of time.

Blue light LED can be helpful in treatment of mild/moderate inflammatory acne. Red light LED, in addition to its anti-aging benefits, has been shown to improve both melasma and psoriasis. It is safe and effective on darker skin types.

IPL treatments, while more painful, typically require far fewer treatments and results are seen more quickly. LED is an excellent choice for someone who has mild/moderate symptoms and is less inclined to choose IPL. As much as LED treatments are indeed effective for treatment of a wide variety of skin concerns, IPL remains superior for clearing hyperpigmentation. LED however, is quite helpful in the treatment of acne and in theory helps with collagen stimulation and healing times.

LED therapy has been gaining some momentum in recent years in the world of medical aesthetics. It certainly holds a solid position therein. IPL, while giving more noticeable results in fewer treatments, may not be for everyone, particularly those with darker skin types. It is important to note that it is suggested that one wear eye protection when using LED, particularly blue light LED which has been shown to be potentially damaging to the retina. Also, speak to your doctor or aesthetician prior to undergoing LED therapy. Explain any medical conditions you may have as well as any medications (such as Accutane and Vitamin A (Retin-A) which may make your skin more sensitive to treatments.

Non-Surgical Fat and Cellulite Reduction

Despite diet and exercise, some areas of the body remain with excess fat. This is very troubling to many. Quite commonly, people see me for non-surgical fat reduction and by outward appearances they really don't appear appreciably overweight. Although you may be in excellent shape, some are genetically predisposed to have areas of their body that resist tightening up. Age is a factor as well. In my 40s it is at least 10 times harder to keep a flat abdomen than what was required in my 20s. Common areas of concern include the abdomen, lower back, upper arms, thighs and the dreaded double chin.

Truthfully, if one were to exercise and diet *enough*, these areas would continue to improve. However, there are many reasons people do not push it to this level. Some may have cardiac issues or arthritis. This makes it both impossible and potentially unsafe to push hard physically. While you may want to be a gym-rat, your body may have a different plan. Others just don't have the time. While these may sound like excuses; that is the reality of the world we live in. 40 hour work weeks are becoming a thing of the past. What happens commonly is that people after months or years of trying to get rid of excess fat ... simply give up. It is incredibly frustrating. Even with an entirely firm body, many still have excess fat in the chin area. This is particularly hard area to reduce, even with a comprehensive diet and wellness plan.

The realm of body contouring continues to grow. Fortunately we have many viable options to help us get rid of excess unwanted fat. Any time I have a consultation with a person in regard to fat reduction, I approach it like I do with many other treatments. If you have an IPL and continue to sunbathe without sunblock, those sunspots are going to come right back. Similarly, if you come in for a fat reduction procedure and do not incorporate a diet and exercise plan into your life, the results in all likelihood are temporary.

The gold standard for reduction of unwanted fat has been liposuction. This procedure can be used to remove fat from just about any area of the body. Chin liposuction as well as abdominal liposuction are procedures well known which have shown fabulous results. The downside of liposuction is that it is an invasive surgical procedure which comes with a higher risk of infection. It is costly and the results are not always perfect either. Occasionally the fat removed is uneven which can result in a distorted result.

There are several different effective technologies available for fat reduction/body contouring. We have already touched on the controlled cooling seen with Coolsculpting to help resolve an unsightly double chin. Coolsculpting and many other technologies can be employed to clear unwanted fat and/or cellulite.

1. **Controlled Cooling** – Coolsculpting
2. **Ultrasound** – Quantashape, Liposonix, Ultrashape
3. **Radiofrequency** – Vanquish RF, Accent XL
4. **Radiofrequency and Infrared** – Velashape
5. **Injection** - Kybella

Fat and Cellulite Reduction Treatments	
Coolsculpting	Controlled Cooling (cryolipolysis)
Quantashape	Ultrasound plus "zonal massage"
Liposonix	High Intensity Focused Ultrasound (HIFU)
Ultrashape	High Intensity Focused Ultrasound (HIFU)
Vanquish RF	Radiofrequency
Accent XL	Radiofrequency
Velashape	Radiofrequency / Infrared / Massage

Controlled Cooling (Cryolipolysis)

Coolsculpting – The Double Chin and More

Earlier we touched on how the Coolsculping Mini will help you lose that double chin. The technology behind Coolsculpting is through 'controlled cooling' (cryolipolysis) of fat cells.

Seven different CoolSculpting attachments are available; each made to treat a different area of the body. It is important to note that while this device indeed does what it claims to, it also typically only results in a 20% fat loss to the treated area per treatment. The average cost for a Coolsculpting procedure is $1000-$1200 with some variation in price based on the size of the area treated. Coolsculpting may require topical anesthetic or pain medication as it is not an entirely painless procedure. The 'freezing' aspect of the procedure offers some anesthesia, however it should be noted that there is a level of discomfort with Coolsculpting.

Ultrasound

I heard an excellent analogy when I first was learning about this technology. Think of ultrasound like a magnifying glass being used to harness sunlight to a focal point where an object (i.e. paper) was to be ignited. Above and below the focal point there is less energy. However, at the focal point there is great energy.

The transducer on the skin releases ultrasound waves in a conical manner with the focal point at about 1.5cm below the surface. When the fat cells are destroyed (liquefied), they break into triglycerides, fatty acids and other debris which is cleared through the lymphatics and liver. Prior to undergoing many of these procedures it is recommended to drink a large amount of water (up to a gallon). In doing so you are helping your lymphatic system and liver clear the broken down fat cells. Results come more quickly when your lymphatic system is well hydrated and working optimally.

Quantashape (Previously Known as VASER SHAPE)

This ultrasound based device also incorporates 'lymphatic zonal massage' into the treatment. Quantashape doesn't exactly destroy the fat cells. It is more accurately described as 'making them leak.' Like other ultrasound fat reduction procedures, drinking a lot of water before and after the procedure is helpful to your lymphatics in clearing of the fat debris. Results are certainly seen after one treatment with optimal results noted following 4-6 treatments.

Liposonix (High Frequency Ultrasound or HIFU)

Liposonix is FDA approved for non-invasive waist circumference reduction. It also uses HIFU. Like other ultrasound treatments, fat cells are permanently destroyed without harming the surface of the skin. Liposonix tends to cause a bit more bruising than what is seen with perhaps Ultrashape. Liposonix treatments are used commonly for fat reduction in the abdomen/saddlebag areas. The maker of the device claims one treatment can reduce your waistline by 1 inch. This translates to a one dress or pant size reduction. There are some results seen immediately, however results continue typically for up to 8 weeks after the procedure.

Ultrashape (High Frequency Ultrasound or HIFU)

This device is FDA approved for abdominal circumference reduction by mechanical disruption of fat cells. It uses high intensity focused ultrasound (HIFU). Ultrashape is described as a very painless procedure. A treatment to the abdomen would take about 30 minutes. One benefit of Ultrashape is that people really *do see* immediate results. It is recommended that patients undergo three treatments spaced two weeks apart. There is no downtime and it is more comfortable than procedures such as Coolsculpting where the 'freezing' of fat cells may be painful.

Radiofrequency (RF)

Radiofrequency is fairly new to the cosmetic industry but has been around for over 70 years. Most recently it has been used for treatment of fat and cellulite. The procedure involves delivery of energy to the deeper skin layers while having no effect on the epidermis. In addition to the fat loss which occurs, collagen remodeling and growth occurs following treatment.

Monopolar vs. Bipolar

There is an important distinction between unipolar (monopolar) and bipolar devices. Monopolar energy travels from the hand-piece to a distant pole, meaning it moves in one direction. Monopolar penetrates the skin to 20mm (deep). This affects both the skin surface and subcutaneous fat. Monopolar is commonly used for skin-tightening to larger areas such as the abdomen, thighs and arms. It is also used for body contouring and cellulite reduction.

Bipolar energy travels in more than one direction from one pole on a hand piece to another and penetrates only 4-5 mm (superficial). Bipolar energy is used for superficial skin tightening.

Vanquish RF

Vanquish utilizes a large panel which lies very close to the skin. It is able to cover a larger area than other devices. It incorporates both unipolar and bipolar RF. Extremes in temperature for periods of time will kill fat cells. Coolsculpting freezes the cells. Vanquish RF heats the fat cells up to 110 degrees which effectively causes them to die. The lymphatics clear the fat cells and debris.

The Accent XL (Alma Lasers)

The accent also uses a combination of unipolar and bipolar radiofrequency to provide heat at different tissue depths. The results from the use of this laser tend to last about 18 months. This laser focuses more on superficial fat and has been shown to be helpful with cellulite. The Accent was featured on the show 'Nip/Tuck." I think of this laser more in terms of how it affects the dermis to make more collagen and elastin. Typically 4-6 treatments are recommended for optimal results.

Velashape III (RF and Infrared)

The Velashape III is a non-invasive body shaping treatment used primarily to treat cellulite and slim the stomach, hip and thigh areas. It uses a combination of technologies (bipolar radiofrequency, infrared, vacuum and massage rollers) for fat and cellulite reduction. People are given an option in some offices as to whether they prefer one long treatment or three shorter treatments.

Lasers That Exfoliate ...And Then Some

Though not nearly as common as traditional chemical peels, lasers do offer an alternative to traditional peels. Some of them peel away layers of the epidermis while others make thousands of tiny 'holes' through the epidermis into the dermis. Some lasers have very little if any effect on the epidermis, focusing more on the underlying dermis. Through the energy being focused on the dermis, there is stimulation of fibroblasts and increased collagen and elastin.

NanoLaserPeel (Sciton) – Epidermal layers removed

This is an erbium-type (resurfacing) laser that uses light energy to instantly remove the top layers of skin. This also accelerates the skin's own renewal process by activating messenger proteins. It offers a more precise way to achieve the exact skin depth desired. Very similar benefits are attained with less downtime than what is seen with a comparable medium depth chemical peel. This procedure was featured on "The Doctors." As the laser is passed over the skin surface, it removes layers of the epidermis. One treatment has been shown to give anti-aging benefits, however as is the case with many lasers, more treatments will give more noticeable and longer-lasting results.

The Halo Laser (Sciton)
Less epidermal damage with deep tissue penetration

Sciton's Halo laser is a hybrid fractional laser. Historically, an ablative laser has long been known as one of the most effective treatments for improving the signs of aging. A true "ablative" laser does extensive damage to the epidermis during the procedure. By causing damage to the outer layers of skin, the skin is forced to heal and increase collagen production. Afterwards the skin continues to tighten and smoothen. Non-ablative lasers 'heat up' the outer layers but don't remove them, hence there is little downtime. The downfall is many treatments are needed to achieve results.

The Halo Laser focuses the energy on the deeper collagen layer (dermis), leaving the surface of your skin with very minimal damage. Hence, in theory, you get the best of both worlds. This is an excellent laser which will improve visible signs of aging including sun damage, uneven skin tone, enlarged pores, fine lines and wrinkles. I highly recommend this laser as an alternative to chemical peels.

Laser Genesis (Cutera)
Focus on the dermis with a reduction in 'diffuse redness'

This treatment achieves results by heating the dermis below the skin surface. Many people have swelling of very tiny vessels in their face commonly in the nose, forehead and cheeks. This results in what is commonly referred to as 'diffuse redness.' This laser heats these vessels to the point where they break down and are ultimately resorbed by the body. Since the dilation of these small capillaries is what is seen with rosacea, this laser treatment has been beneficial in this regard as well. Additionally, since the Laser Genesis exerts much of its effect on the dermis, fibroblasts are stimulated. This results in the promotion of collagen formation. It has also been shown to improve uneven skin texture, tighten pores and reduce fine lines and wrinkles. The laser is moved just above the skin surface and most experience a gentle warming of the skin during the procedure. Immediately after treatment the skin may be slightly red and dark spots (sun damage) will darken and eventually flake off.

Profractional Laser (Sciton)

This profractional laser gives excellent resurfacing results. There is much less downtime here than what is seen with traditional resurfacing treatments that cause more damage to the top layer of skin (epidermis). Profractional makes very narrow channels in the skin covering a mere fraction of the total area of the skin treated. This action initiates the body's wound healing process while leaving the surrounding tissue intact for rapid healing. This type of laser has less patient discomfort and a faster healing time than traditional ablative laser treatments, which cause greater damage to the epidermis.

Clear and Brilliant (Solta Medical)
Millions of holes and more collagen

Clear and Brilliant is a laser which has a small roller attachment. It works through creating millions of tiny superficial treatment columns in the skin which stimulate collagen while also causing a rejuvenated skin surface. The application of antioxidant rich serum after the procedure allows for ingredients to be easily absorbed into the dermis. It improves tone, texture, pores and fine lines.

One thing that should be obvious through reading this chapter is that there are a lot of lasers that can treat literally every skin concern you might have. One issue with laser procedures is that they commonly require several treatments to receive an optimal result. If you go for a Botox or dermal filler injection it typically requires a single treatment. Not so with all lasers. I have had excellent results with the combination of IPL and Fraxel treatments to give powerful anti-aging results. In this scenario there can be a 'one IPL/Fraxel at a time approach.' There are many ways to approach your skin concerns. Lasers are here to stay and the technology keeps improving.

Laser Tattoo Removal

Anyone getting a tattoo certainly feels it is an *awesome* idea at the time. The stark reality is at least 25% of people with tattoos eventually regret having had them done. Johnny Depp had a tattoo professing his love for girlfriend/fiancée Winona Rider stating proudly ... "Winona Forever." When the couple broke up he was left with a bit of a dilemma. "Oh no," thought Johnny, "what now?" His answer was to change the tattoo to read "Wino Forever."

There are other reasons to have a tattoo removed. 40% of those surveyed cited 'employment concerns' as a reason.

There are over 20,000 tattoo parlors in the United States and 14% of all Americans have at least one tattoo. Of those who have had a tattoo, one in ten are either planning to have one removed or have had one removed.

The ink in professional tattoos is injected with a needle through the epidermis into the dermis. Here, the collagen fibers intertwine with the ink-laden dermis making it very difficult to remove the tattoo without damaging any of the surrounding tissue.

Tattoo removal with lasers has been around for 20 years. Like all laser technology, tattoo removal laser options continue to improve every year. Tattoos come in all colors, shapes and sizes and are either done professionally or by 'amateurs.' This wide range dictates that where you go for your tattoo removal should be with someone experienced with these variables.

Lasers Used:

The gold standard for laser tattoo removal has been through the use of a Q-switched laser. This type of laser has the ability to produce light pulses of a higher peak power than a laser operating with a *continuous* output. This property of the laser has been described as having the ability to 'crack' and thereby disrupt the tattoo pigment particles. Although intense pulsed light (IPL) treatments are known to target pigments such as melanin or hemoglobin, they are ineffective with tattoo ink. Some clinics may advertise the use of IPL or non-Q-switched lasers for tattoo removal. My advice would be to steer clear of these places. The clinical data does not support that IPL is safe or effective for tattoo removal.

PicoSure 532nm

Picosure is the latest improvement in tattoo removal technology. The premise here is that the pulse duration here is much shorter, creating a photo-mechanical impact resulting in superior disruption of tattoo ink. While Q-switched lasers use thermal energy to break up the ink particles, PicoSure uses a type of pressure wave technology to shatter the ink into dust-like particles while leaving the surrounding tissue intact. These tiny particles are then cleared and absorbed. PicoSure has shown a strong benefit in the ability to effectively remove tattoos with difficult colors such as red, green, orange and yellow.

The Procedure:

One should have had no UV exposure for a minimum of 4 weeks prior to the procedure. Anesthetic cream may be applied for 20 minutes prior to commencing. Eye protection is recommended and there is commonly a cooling device associated with the use of the laser to keep the skin from becoming too warm and to aid in comfort. The size of the tattoo dictates the length of treatment and may be anywhere from 5 minutes to 1 hour.

Colors:

If you are planning to have a tattoo removal, it will require several treatments. Dark blue and black tattoos tend to respond much better to standard treatment than do colors such as red, green and yellow. PicoSure claims to be able to clear difficult colors such as red, orange and yellow. Amateur tattoos may take between 2-10 treatments (average of 3) to be removed with professional tattoos requiring 5-20 sessions (average of 10). Appointments are typically 4 weeks apart so your tattoo removal journey may take quite a bit longer than it took to have the tattoo in the first place.

Improved laser techniques have allowed more offices to incorporate this service. More young people than ever are getting tattoos and may ultimately regret their decision years down the road. How well a tattoo is removed is related to several important factors.

1. If the tattoo was placed by an amateur or professionally

2. The size of the tattoo

3. The color(s) present.

This is an area of medical aesthetics that is certain to see continued growth with new technologies coming forward at a fairly brisk pace. Many people have considered tattoo removal in the past but have been resistant to move forward. Most felt the tattoo removal procedure would be either too painful or ineffective. Having an unwanted tattoo was perhaps a better option than having a *partially removed* unwanted tattoo.

Like any other medical aesthetic procedure, do your homework. Send an office a picture of your tattoo(s) and hear what options they have for you. Make sure whoever is operating the laser knows what they are doing. Ask to see other 'before and after' pictures from the office you are considering. Keeping these considerations in mind, in all likelihood you will be able to get rid of that unwanted ink.

It is amazing. 20-25 years ago none of the options in this chapter were available. Today people have the privilege of countless choices to treat nearly every cosmetic concern *without surgery*.

As it stands today lasers are able to effectively:

- Clear unwanted brown pigment

- Clear unwanted red discolorations

- Improve skin texture and tone

- Remove hair

- Improve the tightness and contour of just about any place on the face or body

- Reduce fat in multiple areas

- Reduce cellulite

- Exfoliate the skin

- Treat many skin conditions including acne, melasma and rosacea.

- Calm the skin

- Remove tattoos

By the end of this decade (2020) advances will continue to come at a rapid pace. Medical aesthetics procedures bring anti-aging results. This means achieving tangible, youthful and beautiful outcomes with less risk and less downtime than traditional surgical procedures.

Chapter Nine

Skin Types, Skin Diseases & Aging Eyes

The list of available skin care ingredients and aesthetic treatments grows every year. Despite this, many continue to suffer with chronic problematic skin issues and aging eyes.

Acne

70% of young adults between the ages of 12 and 24 have acne. It is the most common skin disorder in the United States affecting 60 million people. While most people think of acne as a teenager problem, it affects 20 million adults as well. The troubling fact is many people with acne fail to seek treatment. Acne begins when the pores of the skin become clogged. Later they may become inflamed and occasionally infected.

Skin cells are continually turning over. The dead cells come to the surface and are shed. This is where the problem with acne starts. On the skin sebaceous glands secrete an oily substance called sebum (see-bum). The sebum normally travels through a tiny hair follicle from the gland to the skin's surface. Sometimes the sebum becomes trapped, mixing with dead skin cells. This causes clogged pores called comedones (come-e-**doh**-neez). A comedone is technically the thick sebum and dead skin cells that block the pore. Bacteria love this environment and grow in the pore, causing redness, inflammation and sometimes infection. This cycle is repeated with acne sufferers.

Blackheads are comedones that reach the skin's surface. Whiteheads are comedones that stay beneath the surface of the skin. The bacterium in the pore can thereby cause small red bumps, pimples, and cysts to develop.

Other factors that contribute are:

1. Changes inside the hair follicle
2. Increased sebum production
3. Changes in the hormone levels (namely the male hormone – androgen, which women have too)
4. Bacteria (*Propionibacterium acne or P. acnes*)
5. Excess keratin in the epidermis known as hyperkeratinization

Acne can cause more than blemishes. The acne itself and resultant scars and dark discolorations lead to many emotional problems. I have seen this commonly in practice. People with acne have a higher incidence of anxiety, depression and low self-esteem.

Treatment Basics:

A search for the term 'acne' on Google results in an overwhelming number of advertisements for products and procedures. There is no shortage of those attempting to sell you a cure for acne. Indeed there are many treatment options but it really comes down to a few key ingredients, patience (6-8 weeks) and repetition. Remember the primary problem is too much sebum and dead skin cells blocking pores.

1. **Salicylic Acid** – Helps to correct the abnormal shedding of cells, unclog pores and prevent lesions. It does not reduce sebum production or kill bacteria. It will exfoliate (remove

dead cells) and is particularly helpful and clearing out pores. Salicylic acid is a *Beta-Hydroxy-Acid.*

2. **Benzoyl Peroxide** – This antibacterial agent gets inside the pore and helps to kill the bacteria. In doing so it also reduces redness and inflammation. It works particularly well on whiteheads.

3. **Hydroquinone** works by decreasing the production and increasing the breakdown of the skin pigment cells (melanosomes). It does this through a complex process of inhibiting an enzyme needed to make melanin.

4. **Alpha Hydroxy Acids** – Work by removing the dead skin cells from the surface of the skin. They can also stimulate collagen and elastin formation in the dermis resulting in tighter and firmer skin.

5. **Over the counter vitamin A** - Studies have shown that even 0.01% retinol has beneficial anti-aging and acne-reducing effects on the skin. Typically over-the-counter preparations come as low (< 0.04%) and medium (0.04-.010%) strengths.

The five ingredients above are all available over the counter; however in severe cases a visit to the dermatologist may be warranted. The ingredients above if used consistently will help clear your acne, but sometimes stronger medicine is needed.

Blue light LED therapy

Blue light therapy penetrates the skin very superficially (approximately 1 mm). However, it has been shown (and FDA approved) to kill the bacteria associated with some forms of acne. This bacterium produces porphyrins as part of its normal metabolism. These porphyrins absorb blue light (and red to a lesser extent) generating reactive oxygen which is toxic to the P. acnes bacteria. Blue light therapy is not a stand-alone treatment for acne. I recommend it when people continue to suffer despite making topical and dietary changes to improve their acne. Both blue and red light can be used concomitantly to treat acne. Blue light, as noted though its ability to clear bacteria; Red light through action on a cellular level help reduce inflammation and hasten skin healing.

Blue light, while clearly a means to improve mild to moderate inflammatory acne, is far less affective for cystic acne, blackheads and whiteheads.

Essential Oils

When I was in medical school in the early 90s there was really no discussion about alternative measures to cure common illnesses or skin conditions. The thought process was just not there. Antibiotics for acne were a common first line treatment. Through my study of dermatology and skin care it became clear to me that there are many options to consider when treating acne or other skin concerns. Antibiotics should be an absolute last resort and ideally should never be used at all.

25 years ago the Medical Journal of Australia showed that 5% tea tree oil was as effective as 5% benzoyl peroxide in a study of 124 patients. Tea tree oil worked more slowly to reduce open and closed comedones, but also had fewer side effects than benzoyl peroxide. This is a non-comedogenic beauty oil and is beneficial in the treatment of mild to moderate inflammatory acne.

Jojoba oil contains vitamin E, B-complex, copper and zinc. Jojoba oil closely resembles human sebum (the substance made by sebaceous glands). Why use an oil to treat acne that mirrors sebum? Jojoba oil tricks the skin into thinking there is more than enough sebum. Hence, the skin actually *produces less sebum*. Jojoba oil helps clear the skin and open clogged pores. It brings antibacterial properties vs. acne bacteria. Jojoba oil very non-allergenic and is helpful particularly with dry or sensitive skin types as well.

Review of Comedogenesis

Comedogenesis is best defined simply as "the tendency to clog pores." Essential oils are not typically at the forefront of discussions in regard to acne care. However, the use of these oils has become very commonplace. They can have either positive or negative effects on acne. The table we saw earlier needs to be revisited here. Middle aged women in particular may develop adult onset acne.

COMEDOGENESIS

Non-Comedogenic	Mildly Comedogenic	Moderately Comedogenic	Most Comedogenic
Argan Oil	Calendula Oil	Almond Oil	Cocoa Butter
Marula Oil	Jojoba Oil *	Apricot Oil	**Coconut Oil**
Tea Tree Oil *	Chamomile Oil	Avocado Oil	Corn Oil
Hemp Seed Oil	Emu Oil	Olive Oil	Flaxseed Oil
Safflower Oil	Grape Seed Oil	Peanut Oil	Mink Oil
Sunflower Oil	Pomegranate Oil	Primrose Oil	Soybean Oil
Mineral Oil	Rosehip Oil	Sesame Oil	Wheat Germ Oil

Better for acne – Tea Tree Oil and Jojoba Oil

Case Study: I cared for a woman who presented with adult onset acne. After trying many over the counter remedies she came to see me. She continued to exclaim, "I have no idea where this is coming from. I have changed 'nothing' in my skin care for 20 years!" Her skin care regimen was excellent as was her skin. In fact she looked perhaps 10 years younger than her stated age. She used cleansers, hyaluronic moisturizers and was very good about UV protection. Ultimately we found out that she was always finishing her daily regimen with a light coating of coconut oil. In the following weeks we discontinued coconut oil and began substituting it with tea tree oil. I also added the use of a salicylic acid cleanser, microdermabrasion and blue light therapy. Within 2 months her skin was totally clear.

Hence, I will reiterate the importance of comedogenesis with the use of essential oils here. If you suffer from acne, tea tree oil or jojoba oil are two excellent choices.

When to see the doctor:

I recommend seeing a doctor if the over the counter treatments do not work or you are not satisfied with the results you are getting. The doctor can prescribe:

1. A higher strength salicylic acid or benzoyl peroxide
2. An antibiotic in the form of a cream or a pill you take by mouth
3. A Retinol, such as Retin-A or Renova (see table)
4. In severe cases the doctor may prescribe a Retinol to take by mouth (Accutane). This needs to be prescribed by a doctor very familiar with this drug. Patients need to be monitored for signs of toxicity while taking Accutane.

Prescription Vitamin A	Powerful form of Vitamin A	Primary Uses
Retin- A	Tretinoin	Acne
Renova	Tretinoin	Sun damage/ Anti-aging
Tri-Luma	Tretinoin (and hydroquinone)	Sun damage / Anti-aging
Tazorac	Tazarotene	Acne / Anti-aging
Differin	Adapalene	Acne / Anti-aging

Treatment of Acne Scarring or Pigment Changes:

One of the most troubling problems with acne is the cumulative damage it does to the skin. After the acne has cleared, redness, pigment changes and scarring may persist. Topical treatments, exfoliation, the use of lasers, microneedling and dermal filler injections can help you to make huge improvements in these issues related to chronic acne.

1. Topical Treatments

a. Vitamin C-Ester

This vitamin has strong anti-inflammatory qualities which stimulate the skin to produce more collagen and elastin. If used regularly it will also help to fade dark spots and smoothen out inconsistencies in skin pigment.

b. Vitamin E

Vitamin E is a powerful topical antioxidant which has been shown to offer a favorable outcome in the treatment of scars. It also helps to fade unwanted pigment. Vitamin E is not recommended when acne is active. However, as a topical agent to help treat the sequelae of chronic acne, it is an excellent choice.

c. Alpha lipoic acid

Alpha lipoic acid's antioxidant and anti-aging effects help to improve skin texture and tone. The anti-inflammatory effects of alpha lipoic acid have been shown to be beneficial in different causes of skin inflammation. Many with changes due to acne have areas of persistent redness. Here alpha lipoic acid is particularly beneficial.

2. Exfoliation

People with skin issues due to acne can reap great benefits through both physical and chemical exfoliation. A medium strength chemical peel is very effective at clearing unwanted pigment or skin tone inconsistencies. A Jessner's peel which is a combination of three ingredients (resorcinol, salicylic acid and glycolic acid) has been shown to be very beneficial in both the treatment of acne and acne scarring.

3. Laser Procedures

The good news is lasers offer many options in your quest to clear the scarring and/or pigment changes that years of acne have caused to your skin. The gold standard for clearing unwanted pigment is intense pulsed light (IPL). These treatments will target melanin, disrupt it and clear it. In terms of laser alternatives to improve acne scars my choice is Fraxel skin resurfacing. Here thousands of holes are made in the epidermis, into the dermis to form an entirely new surface while powerfully stimulating collagen and elastin formation in the dermis.

There are other laser procedures we have discussed including NanoLaserPeel, the Halo Laser and Clear + Brilliant. These lasers give similar results to a medium chemical peel, and more. They have less downtime than medium peels while doing a fabulous job of clearing pigment and improving the texture and tone of the skin.

4.   Microneedling

Microneedling is an excellent alternative to laser skin resurfacing and comes with less downtime. It can be used on any skin type and does an excellent job of remodeling the skin surface. Much like Fraxel, microneedling gives an improved skin surface while aggressively stimulating collagen and elastin in the dermis. To improve acne scarring you really need to improve the collagen and elastin beneath the epidermis as well as the epidermal layer itself. With this procedure, ingredients such as platelet rich plasma (PRP) can be placed on the skin surface during the procedure. As the needles penetrate the skin, so does the PRP. This is a powerful means to help resolve acne scarring. I highly recommend microneedling with PRP for treatment of acne scarring and for its ant-aging benefits.

5.   Red Light LED

This treatment was discussed as helpful in the treatment of acne (along with blue light LED). However, red light LED will also help to remove unwanted pigment and increase collagen in the dermis.

6.   Dermal Fillers

While certainly not a first line treatment for acne scarring, the use of dermal fillers can be quite helpful when larger scars (or 'pock marks') are present. The best dermal fillers to use are those with a low G-prime and smaller particle size. My dermal filler choices for treatment of acne scarring are Restylane Silk or Belotero. In the hands of an experienced injector, these dermal fillers will plump up the scarred areas nicely. The injection itself also helps stimulate fibroblasts to help produce more collagen and elastin as well.

Dos and Don'ts:

- If you play a sport, particularly one that involves wearing a helmet, be aware. As you sweat, the sebaceous glands secrete more sebum. When there is pressure on these areas from a helmet, it increases the likelihood of blocked pores. Make sure you are washing with a salicylic acid cleanser to clear sebum, exfoliate and keep those pores clear.
- Touch your face as little as possible. The oil on your hands does nothing but increase what is already an excess amount of oil (sebum) on your skin.
- While I know this may be a challenge, don't pick at your skin. It is better to let the skin heal naturally.
- Be gentle with your face. Do not scrub, this just irritates your face and makes your skin produce more oil/sebum. When you wash your face use your fingertips, don't scrub aggressively with sponge or washcloth.
- If you have oily hair, make sure you shampoo regularly.

When people think of acne, their first thoughts are related to what they can place on or *do to* their skin. For many it's creams, lotions, benzoyl peroxide, blue light or laser treatments. What far too many neglect is the fact that certain dietary measures can make a world of difference in the treatment and management of acne.

Acne Diet

In 1826 Anthelme Brillat-Savarin said "Tell me what you eat and I will tell you what you are." Translation: "You are what you eat." My aunt used to say it all the time and she had beautiful skin.

Without a doubt, topical preparations are extraordinarily helpful at getting rid of dead skin cells, opening pores and reducing inflammation. I have had fantastic results using lasers as well. As a teenage acne sufferer myself, I knew without a doubt that different foods made it worse. Like any difficult and chronic skin condition, we have to attack it from every possible angle. The Clear Skin diet translates beautifully for the treatment of acne (and rosacea).

To Review:

1. Water

You lose water through sweat, breathing, the urinary, and the intestinal tract. I encourage all acne sufferers to drink at least 64 – 80 ounces of water per day. When the skin is dry, secretions are thicker and pores are more easily blocked. Adequate hydration is a good idea for anyone. With acne-prone skin it is *imperative*.

2. Green Leafy Vegetables

Those with acne need foods loaded with antioxidants and vitamin A. Arugula, kale, collard greens, Brussel sprouts, romaine lettuce and spinach are high in vitamin A (and chlorophyll). Anything with vitamin A is going to be helpful to combat acne and regenerate the skin. Other foods with vitamin A include carrots, papaya, tomatoes, watermelon and apricots. Fluctuations in hormones trigger breakouts. The green leafy vegetables in this food group help to stabilize these.

3. Vitamin A and C-rich Fruits

These foods include oranges, kiwi, papaya, lemon, cantaloupe, strawberries, blueberries and bananas. They are all high in antioxidants and vitamins A and C. Vitamin A is a natural anti-acne vitamin and helps regenerate new skin. Vitamin C fights free radicals, increases collagen and reduces wrinkles.

4. Omega 3 Fatty Acid-Rich Seafood (Salmon, Tuna, Lobster, Crab, Shrimp)

These fatty acids help at the level of the individual cell by improving the health of the cell membrane, giving the skin a healthy glow and improved skin texture. Certain components of seafood may also have anti-bacterial qualities and help protect against UVA/UVB rays. Omega 3 fatty acids are also found in walnuts, canola oil and flax seed.

5.   Green Tea, Nuts & Legumes

My favorites include green beans, pinto beans, chickpeas, walnuts and almonds. Green tea is loaded with antioxidants and fights inflammation. Nuts and legumes are high in vitamin E which brings antioxidant power as well.

6.   Limit High Glycemic Index Foods

I realize there are many high glycemic index foods and avoiding them altogether is a very tall order. My first goal with acne sufferers is to *limit* these. When high glycemic index foods are consumed there is a sharp rise in the sugar level in the bloodstream. This is quickly followed by insulin release. The insulin spike leads to hormone fluctuations and breakouts. These foods include white rice, sugary cereals, potatoes, French fries, pretzels, scones, muffins, Coca-Cola/Pepsi. These are the most common offenders. Fried food is problematic as well.

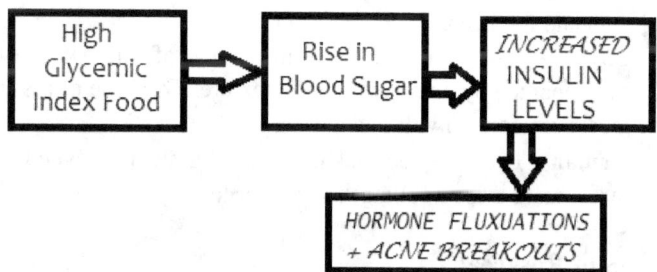

Fighting acne requires a multifaceted approach. These Clear Skin (and acne) dietary guidelines are aimed at helping your skin become clear and vibrant. While they may be tough to follow exactly, it should give you something to refer to when you or someone you care about suffers from acne. The closer you are able to follow these dietary guidelines, the clearer your skin will be. That I guarantee.

Rosacea

Rosacea affects over 45 million people worldwide. Its rash typically presents as flushing and redness affecting the cheeks, nose and forehead but may also involve the neck, chest, back, scalp or ears. Left untreated, rosacea can worsen with more permanent symptoms including continuous facial redness, red bumps, eye irritation, burning or stinging sensations and the presence of small blood vessels near the skin surface. Rosacea can be triggered by many factors and may be confused with acne, allergic dermatitis or other skin diseases.

Types of Rosacea:

Rosacea can be categorized into four main types. These are based on the blemishes/lesions seen on the skin and the areas involved.

1. **Erythremato-telangectasic** – This essentially means redness with visible blood vessels. It is many times associated with a stinging or burning sensation.
2. **Papulopustular** – Redness and swelling with papules and pustules, similar to acne. It is commonly seen on the cheeks, chin and forehead.
3. **Phymatous** – Here there is thickening of the skin itself accompanied by a red and bumpy texture. This type of rosacea most commonly involves the nose.
4. **Ocular** – Eyes are red and irritated with swollen eyelids. In many cases these swellings are similar to a stye.

Causes of Rosacea:

Rosacea was originally thought to have an unknown origin. However, most experts agree that this skin disorder is related to blood vessels in the dermis suffering damage due to certain stimuli. Small vessels stay dilated too long or remain permanently dilated. As a result, the body sends immune and inflammatory cells to the area which contributes to the resulting redness, pustules and papules seen.

I try to explain rosacea as a type of skin allergy. However, it is not an allergic dermatitis per se. When you consider that some people have a more severe allergic reaction to bee stings, similarly, those with rosacea have a more pronounced skin reaction to certain skin triggers more so than the average population. Put another way, people with rosacea seem to have an exaggerated response similar to an 'allergy' to certain factors. This allergy results in the skin changes seen.

Like many chronic medical illnesses (and I consider this an 'illness'), this appears to have a genetic component. It is more common in fair skinned individuals, middle aged women and those of European or Celtic descent.

Triggers:

Triggers are the most important consideration in the treatment of rosacea.

Every person being treated for rosacea should keep a skin diary.

Like any chronic, recurrent skin disease, rosacea requires a multifaceted approach. Identification of exacerbating factors is necessary to move forward with treatment. There is no way to give an all-inclusive list of potential rosacea triggers. When I have patients keep a skin diary, I ask them to document when their skin appears worse paying particular attention to the following:

- Foods – particularly hot or spicy foods
- Sun (UVA/UVB) exposure
- Stress – either emotional stress or physical stress (exercise)
- Hot showers or baths
- Alcohol consumption
- Medications, particularly steroid, hormone or blood pressure medicines (Steroids should never be used to treat rosacea)
- A change in bed sheets, detergents, dryer sheets, shampoos, cleansers, body lotions or creams
- Skin care ingredients containing strong perfumes / alcohol
- Presence of menopausal symptoms

- Relationship to menstrual cycles.

Treatment:

I like to divide treatment of rosacea into five categories. The order in which I attack rosacea is: **triggers, diet, skin care, laser treatments and medicines.**

1. **Triggers** – Based on the skin diary, avoidance of triggers is of paramount importance. Every rosacea patient *has* and needs to *identify* triggers. They are an all-important preventative measure. However, avoidance of triggers, while helpful, does not typically cause a full resolution of rosacea symptoms.

2. **Diet** – Anti-oxidant rich fruits and vegetables such as broccoli, Brussel sprouts and cantaloupe are excellent sources of dietary anti-oxidants. The Clear Skin diet, which includes foods high in anti-oxidants and fish with omega 3 fatty acids, is helpful in the treatment of acne *and rosacea*.

3. **Skin Care** – This is a vital category in the treatment of rosacea. The skin is an amazing organ. It protects us every day from perpetual environmental insults and has an amazing ability to heal itself. As I have mentioned, those with rosacea have skin that is hyper-sensitive to environmental stimuli. After identification and avoidance of triggers where possible and making positive dietary adjustments, the next focus is on skin care. This is aimed at helping the skin heal without giving the body (and the person) potential side effects and complications of more aggressive treatments.

   - **Alpha Lipoic Acid** – This ingredient carries with it outstanding antioxidant and anti-inflammatory power. A benefit of using alpha lipoic acid is that it helps other antioxidants work more efficiently.

- **Other anti-oxidants** – Skin care regimens which include vitamin A (retinol), vitamin E, Vitamin C and Vitamin C-ester are quite helpful.
- **Polyphenols** – From grape seed, green tea or olive oil
- **Niacinamide** – Has been shown to improve the skin's barrier function resulting in a diminished reaction to irritants in patients with rosacea.
- Other ingredients include gamma linoleic acid, burdock root (anti-inflammatory and anti-bacterial) and fish oil (omega 3 fatty acids).

4. **Laser Treatments** – While understandably controversial, I have seen improvement of rosacea symptoms through the use of lasers. Intense pulsed light in wavelengths targeting tiny blood vessels under the skin is helpful in many cases. It typically requires a minimum of 3-6 treatments to achieve optimal results.

5. **Medications** – Topical or oral medication may be used in severe cases and certainly is helpful to many. It is not my preferred initial treatment. The list of medications for rosacea is long as are the possible side effects associated with them.

- **Blood pressure medications**

   Medicines that lower the blood pressure including clonidine and beta blockers may be helpful. They appear to have an overall calming effect as well as a direct effect on the blood vessels. These medications can be associated with side effects including drowsiness or dizziness.

- **Isotretinoin**

   This has been used to treat acne in severe cases and has also been used (in lower doses) to treat rosacea. Limited studies have shown this medication's ability to bring tangible results in the long-term treatment of rosacea. I am not a fan of isotretinoin for acne or rosacea. It requires monitoring of blood tests to assure the medication is not toxic to the liver.

- **Antibiotics**

  These may be taken by mouth or applied topically to the skin. These include tetracycline, doxycycline, clindamycin and metronidazole amongst others. Antibiotics have been shown to help some cases but should never be a 'stand-alone' treatment for rosacea (or acne). In fact, experts agree that any positive effect that an antibiotic has on rosacea has more to do with the antibiotic's *anti-inflammatory properties* than its anti-bacterial properties.

Rosacea affects millions and sufferers really need a systematic, safe and simple approach to getting their rosacea treated and *kept under control*. A long term cure requires simple daily steps. I begin with a skin diary and the right diet. The next step is the use of alpha lipoic acid and anti-oxidants both by mouth and topically. In certain cases intense pulsed light has proven helpful but may take 3-6 treatments for optimal results. Finally, antibiotics and other medications may be used in severe and resistant cases. In my opinion medications should really be used only in the cases resistant to conservative measures and never as a first line treatment.

Melasma

Melasma is a condition of the skin where brown spots or blotches appear on areas of the face. These commonly appear on the cheeks, nose, chin, forehead and lips. The brown areas can be irregularly shaped or have a smooth border. They develop gradually over time. Their presence is triggered primarily by hormones and UVA/UVB rays; both of which ultimately cause an increased production of the pigment *melanin.* Melasma is also known as 'Chloasma' or 'Mask of Pregnancy.'

What causes Melasma?

The melanin pigment in the upper skin layer (epidermis) is stimulated by certain factors. The hormonal nature of this skin condition makes it more present in women however melasma can be present in men as well.

1. Estrogen and Progesterone (hormones)

- During pregnancy, fluctuations in the levels of these hormones may cause areas of the face to darken. Regardless of a woman's age during pregnancy this may occur. Those pregnant in summer months or in warm climates where there is potential for increased UV ray exposure are at greater risk. If melasma starts during pregnancy, it will frequently resolve after delivery.
- Oral contraceptives also contain these hormones and may result in the development of melasma. If this condition occurs, it is typically within the first 1-3 months after the medication is begun.
- Hormone replacement therapy. Women choose hormone replacement for a variety of reasons at and after menopause. Even though a woman may not have suffered from melasma during pregnancy, she may develop melasma at the age of menopause when she begins hormone replacement therapy.

2. UVA/UVB Rays

With exposure from these damaging rays, the skin increases melanin production, making it darker in an attempt to prevent further damage. In those prone to melasma, the UV rays can make these hyperpigmented areas darker and larger. Anyone with a history of melasma needs to be certain to protect themselves from UV rays.

3. Darker Skin Types / Genetic

While melasma can affect any skin type, it is present to a greater degree in those with darker skin types. If your mother had melasma during pregnancy, while on oral contraceptives or while taking hormone replacement therapy, you are more likely to develop melasma as well.

4. Thyroid Disease

Those with thyroid disease have been shown to have an increased incidence of melasma. While melasma rarely is the first symptom of thyroid disease, those with new onset of melasma at any age should have a blood test to check levels of thyroid hormone. Similarly, it is imperative that those with thyroid disease who suffer from melasma be treated optimally.

Diagnosis of Melasma

Melasma has a very distinct pattern on the face, so it is typically diagnosed on appearance alone. The brown areas are of different shapes and sizes with some areas darker than others. Some areas have a smooth border while others are irregular. To confirm the diagnosis, a doctor may use a Wood's Lamp which helps demonstrate the presence and pattern of excess pigment in the epidermis.

The good news is there are many effective preventative and treatment measures for rosacea.

Preventing Melasma

1. Women who are taking oral contraceptives can speak with their doctor in regard to taking an alternate medication with a lower concentration (dosage) of estrogen and/or progesterone *or* consider an alternative form of contraception (i.e. intra-uterine device).

2. Women taking hormone replacement therapy may speak with their doctor about taking a lower, yet effective, dosage. Taking

the medication in the evening so the peak levels are present during the night vs. during the daylight hours has been helpful to some women.

3. Sunblock! Those who are pregnant, taking oral contraceptives or on hormone replacement therapy should be aggressive about using sunblock containing titanium oxide or zinc oxide with an SPF of 50 to block damaging UV rays. In addition, wearing a sun hat is a great idea as well.

4. Stress: One thing I have learned in over 20 years as a physician is that stress makes *everything worse*. Medical conditions like hypertension, diabetes and heart disease as well as skin problems like acne, eczema, psoriasis and melasma can be exacerbated by stress. Taking time for yoga, exercise, mediation, reading or whatever activity (or lack of activity) that you choose to help relax ... will help your skin.

Treating Melasma

1. **Bleaching Creams -** These do not actually 'bleach' the skin. Rather, they reduce the production of melanin ultimately resulting in less pigment visible on the skin. The gold standard in this category is hydroquinone. Depending on the country in which you live different strengths of hydroquinone are available over the counter (OTC). In the US Hyrdoquinone 2% is available OTC. Due to the fact that this product is blocking melanin production it makes your skin more likely to burn. It should not be used in pregnant or nursing women and typically for no more than 6 months. People with allergic disorders like eczema, psoriasis or asthma should only use hydroquinone (of any strength) under the care of a doctor. Avoid the nose and eyes. Doctors can prescribe higher concentrations of 4-10% in particularly difficult cases.

2. **Tretinoin (Vitamin A)** – In certain individuals, the use of vitamin A preparations, due to their ability to increase cell

turnover, can help fade the brown discolorations of melasma. Tretinoin also cannot be used in pregnant or nursing women.

3. **Microdermabrasion** – Whether it is an aluminum oxide or diamond tip system, this means of physical exfoliation is helpful to melasma sufferers. Some machines can allow for solutions of exfoliating acids like salicylic acid (which also clears pores) to be infused into the skin during the procedure. Typically these procedures are most effective if repeated every 3-4 weeks. Once symptoms are improved and controlled microdermabrasion should continue every 6-8 weeks.

4. **Chemical Peels** – Glycolic acid is the best known agent used for chemical peels. Peels should be done by an aesthetician or a physician well trained with their application. The acid is placed onto the skin for a period of time. The goal is the removal of the top layer (epidermis) of skin. Chemical peels are an effective means to help clear away unwanted pigment along with helping to rejuvenate the skin and clear pores.

5. **Lasers** – It is important to understand that any laser procedure used for treatment of melasma should be done by someone well versed in the use of lasers. Intense Pulsed Light (IPL), though helpful with other types of sun damage, can make melasma worse so should not be used. The Fraxel laser is FDA approved for treatment of melasma and has shown the best results. A Fraxel laser breaks the light into small fragments (or pixels). This provides an effective treatment for melasma without the long downtime that you may experience with a more aggressive chemical peel.

Other Measures to Consider

1. Apple Cider Vinegar. The citric acid present here can help to fade pigment. Equal amounts of apple cider vinegar and water are applied to the pigmented areas and allowed to dry, then

rinsed with lukewarm water. There are those who have had fantastic results with this approach but there are typically better alternatives. Since, in effect, you are applying a mild acid to the skin, the use of apple cider vinegar is essentially similar to performing a very light chemical peel.

2. **Niacinamide (Vitamin B3)** Niacinamide is one of my favorite vitamins for the skin. It improves skin elasticity, has anti-inflammatory properties and helps block the transfer of pigment to skin cells. It also has the ability to block UVA/UVB rays.

A Consistent Approach

Treatment of melasma, like any chronic skin condition, can be a challenge. However, with a systematic and consistent approach you will get results.

1. Wear a hat and SPF vs. UVA/UVB of 50.
2. Try hydroquinone or tretinoin if you are not pregnant or nursing
3. Consider a series of microdermabrasion or chemical peels or even apple cider vinegar.
4. If you can afford it, consider a Fraxel laser treatment.
5. Speak with your doctor to determine if your estrogen/progesterone-containing medication can be changed to a lower (yet still effective) dose.

Dry Skin

Your skin protects you from continual environmental insults. UVA and UVB rays, wind, cold, moisture, viruses, bacteria and an endless array of irritants including molds, dust and pollen are around your skin constantly. These may leave your skin itchy, dry, red, and in severe cases may result in dermatitis, eczema, psoriasis or infection. Your skin is an amazing organ and powerful barrier to the external environment. Taking care of your skin will keep this barrier, smooth, strong, well hydrated and looking good.

I believe there to be four skin types. These are normal, dry, oily and sensitive. These are skin types and not diseases. People also do not necessarily have the same skin type at all times. A person who has had normal skin through many years living in the Midwest may suddenly have dry skin after moving to the Nevada desert.

Practical Advice for Dry Skin:

1. Changes in Humidity

This happens when there is a change in the moisture of the air surrounding us. This problem occurs most commonly in the winter months. Once it gets colder, people turn on their heaters. While heating your home, moisture levels drop appreciably. The result is commonly a comfortable yet dry home … and dry skin. Our skin loves moisture and when there is not enough in the environment the skin becomes dry and itchy.

Keep your home between 67 and 70 degrees and use a humidifier. Ideal humidity in the home is 45-55%. The cold air outside does nothing to help, so cover up sensitive areas. Wear gloves to protect your hands, lip balm and a scarf to protect your face from damaging cold, wind and snow.

2. Showers

There are many ways to either help or hurt your skin with your daily shower (or bath). To begin, staying in a very hot shower for extended periods of time can strip away natural oils from your skin. These natural oils help keep your skin soft and moist. While hot steamy showers may make your muscles feel better, they are damaging to your skin. Showers should be brief, and with cooler water. If you are regularly fogging up the mirrors in your bathroom, you are likely taking showers that are too hot or too long (or both). When in the shower, avoid scrubbing your skin. The premise is the same, scrubbing does nothing but strip away protective oils. Use your hands or a very soft washcloth in the shower to prevent excess skin dryness or irritation. Finally when drying off after a shower, don't scrub ... simply pat dry. You should ideally have some moisture left on your skin after your shower. When your skin is damp it is an ideal time to use a moisturizer.

3. Hydrate your Face

Using products containing hyaluronic acid, dimethicone or glycerin are very helpful here. SPF of 20 or more is a fantastic idea as well. This way you are not only protecting your face and helping to keep moisture in, but you are also blocking damaging UVA/UVB rays.

4. Soaps

Many ingredients in soaps or shampoos have harsh chemicals or perfumes which can be irritating to your skin, so pick carefully. All too commonly a patient presents to my office with a new rash or very dry irritated skin, only to find out it was due to some new soap he/she was using. Using unscented soaps or gentle cleansers is preferable for the cleansing of your skin.

5. Other Skin Irritants

Do not neglect to realize that clothing, bed sheets, necklaces, watches, rings or dryer sheets are potential irritants to your skin. Wool and polyester are more prone to cause skin irritation than cotton or natural fabrics.

6. More Serious Problems

If your skin continues to be dry, itchy, red, and blotchy or cracked it may indicate a more serious problem such as dermatitis, eczema, psoriasis or even infection. Certain medical conditions such as diabetes, hypothyroidism and lupus can also first appear as a rash that does not resolve. If this is the case you should see a dermatologist. There are many topical creams, lotions, shampoos or even oral medication that can be prescribed to help.

Using the Right Products for Dry Skin

Dry skin can also be caused by products you put on the skin such as a cleanser that is too harsh or a moisturizer that doesn't quite keep the skin moist enough.

If you have dry skin, use a gentle cleanser. A beauty bar containing emollients such as lanolin or olive oil is an excellent choice as well.

When using a moisturizer, you need the ingredients that are the most hydrating. Products with glycerin, dimethicone or hyaluronic acid are very hydrating while also slowing the loss of moisture from the skin surface. Beauty oils effectively trap moisture in the skin. Olive oil and coconut oil are two examples which can be used in those without acne. If your skin is acne-prone, choose sunflower, jojoba or wheat germ oil. Other skin care ingredients to strongly consider with dry skin include niacinamide and alpha lipoic acid. Cosmetic products that are labeled *nourishing, moisturizing or hydrating* are typically oil based and are better choices for dry skin.

Dry Skin Checklist

1. Avoid harsh soaps, grainy cleansers or buffing pads.
2. Select moisturizers formulated with glycerin, dimethicone or hyaluronic acid which help moisturize and keep moisture in.
3. Apply moisturizer when your face is still damp to help keep as much moisture as you can 'beneath' the moisturizer.
4. Use a gentle cleanser.
5. Keep your showers brief and cool.
6. Keep your home's humidity at a level that will not make your skin overly dry (ideally 45-55%).
7. Make sure you are wearing SPF 20+ on face, neck and hands to prevent the drying effects of UV rays.

Oily Skin

Oily skin (Seborrhea) is caused by excess skin oil (sebum). This is a daily annoyance affecting men and women of any age. Commonly products claiming to eliminate oily skin contain ingredients which irritate your skin ultimately triggering more oil production. In the long term this simply makes matters worse.

Around the age of puberty, increased hormone levels (androgens – present in males and females) cause increased oil production. The oiliness seems to subside after puberty but in some it persists or even worsens in adulthood. Changes in hormone levels during pregnancy may also contribute. Many times the skin becomes oilier during certain seasons, particularly when it is more humid. On one hand, those with excess skin oil tend to age better. On the negative side, people with oily skin may have thickening of pore lining, which prevents oil (sebum) from flowing out properly. This can lead to blackheads, white or clear bumps and acne.

People with oily skin know and are familiar with the daily struggle that occurs with this skin type. There are certain characteristics those with oily skin experience:

1. The face feels comfortable and moist for an hour or two after cleansing, however by mid-day begins to feel oily.
2. Applying makeup is difficult at times.
3. The more oily areas of the face have blackheads, white or clear bumps, or acne.
4. The pores are visibly enlarged, especially on the nose, chin, and forehead (T-zone).
5. The oily areas are more present in this T-zone.

Oily Skin Care Plan

Products that feel like they are drying to your skin may feel good but they typically make matters worse by ultimately causing your skin to produce more oil. The first step in caring for oily skin is to take a critical look at your current skin-care routine.

Your skin care regimen to control oily skin needs to be simple yet effective. Follow a plan which includes cleansing, exfoliating, toning and hydrating your skin. This will result in less oil, smaller pores and fewer breakouts.

1. Cleanse:

Use a gentle facial cleanser twice a day. Dermatologists are in full agreement that cleansing the skin is the best way to reduce oil. Make sure your cleanser is non-alkaline (i.e. don't use soaps in bar form). The goal here is to clean your skin without stripping and irritating it. Fragrance-free products containing benzoyl peroxide, salicylic acid or glycolic acid are often considered best. These are slightly acidic so start off with only a small amount to make sure your skin doesn't have an adverse reaction. Wash and rinse your face with lukewarm water, not hot. Hot water simply irritates your skin.

2. Tone

Use an *alcohol free* toner with ingredients like alpha hydroxy acids. A good skin toner helps skin heal, shrinks large pores and reduces inflammation through clearing traces of dead skin cells or makeup that can lead to clogged pores.

3. Exfoliate

Exfoliation is one of the most important skin-care steps for oily skin. This skin type tends to have an extra-thick layer of built-up dead skin cells on the surface of the skin, along with a thickened pore lining. Exfoliation is the best way to remove dead cells and unclog pores. Those who exfoliate regularly have skin that is softer and smoother.

The best exfoliating ingredient for oily skin is salicylic acid; it exfoliates not only the surface of your skin but also inside the pore lining, thus improving pore function and allowing oil to flow easily to the surface. Salicylic acid brings anti-inflammatory properties as well. In addition, ideally your exfoliant or toner will contain hydroquinone which over time will help fade dark discolorations from past blemishes.

4. Sun Protection and Hydration

It may seem odd that you need to moisturize and hydrate skin that is already oily but even those with oily skin need moisture and UV ray protection. If your skin is exposed to UVA or UVB rays it can aggravate and irritate your skin; producing more oil. Ideally you want to moisturize with a lightweight liquid, lotion, serum or gel that has a minimum of SPF 20. Even if you have oily skin, sunblock is essential for preventing wrinkles and reducing skin discolorations.

5. Absorb Excess Oil

As you begin to get your oily skin under control, it's likely that you still will need to use products that absorb oil on a weekly, biweekly or even daily basis. Many find the use of blotting papers very helpful. This is a quick, effective solution to soak up excess oil. They won't cut down on your skin's oil production though, so this treatment should be paired with a cleansing regimen for the best results

Clearing oily skin is well within your reach if you follow a simple straightforward plan and avoid common pitfalls that may further irritate the skin and increase oil production.

Combination Skin

It would appear to me as though the term 'combination skin' may have fully run its course. I am at a crossroads as to whether or not this term is of help to anyone. With no hesitation, I agree that some people have more oil on certain parts of their face than others. However, nobody's face has a perfectly symmetric and equally distributed pattern of sebaceous (oil) glands. Most everyone has more oil glands through the T-zone area (forehead, brow, nose and/or chin). Does that mean everyone has combination skin? If everyone has combination skin, how can we describe it a specific skin 'type'? A definition often heard is, "When two or more skin types appear on the face at the same time." The definition seems benign enough. Why question it?

WebMD says, "A combination skin type can be dry or normal in some areas and oily in others, such as the T-zone." Since technically everyone has more oil glands in the T-zone, aren't they basically saying some people have dry, normal or oily skin? They continue by identifying 'shiny skin and blackheads' as commonplace with combination skin. What? *Shiny skin* points to combination skin? People with blackheads in the T-zone area need to consider treatment for acne which is a skin *disease* not a skin *type*.

Skin Types

1. People who have <u>oily skin</u> may produce more oil on their entire face and the T-zone area.
2. People who have <u>dry skin</u> may produce less oil on their entire face and the T-zone area.
3. People with <u>normal skin</u> may produce an average amount of oil on their entire face, yet still tend to have more oil in the T-zone area.

I have mentioned I believe there to be four skin types; normal, dry, oily and sensitive.

It also may appear as though sensitive skin and combination skin have a large overlap. Everyone's skin is sensitive to some degree and clearly some have *more* sensitive skin. I might suggest that those with sensitive skin are also prone to having varying degrees of moisture and/or oiliness on different areas of their face.

What if someone has normal skin, but has an extra oily T-zone. Perhaps this is combination skin. In colder climates, people turn on their heaters in the winter and the humidity drops. This results in lower moisture in the air and the skin. Now someone with normal skin has dry skin. Someone prone to acne on their cheeks may scrub/exfoliate that area aggressively. They may have started with normal skin, but now have dry skin on their cheeks, an oily T-zone and normal skin elsewhere. Is that combination skin? Someone may use a large amount of irritating skin care products resulting in dry patches, oily patches and normal patches. Is that combination skin, or is that a patchy allergic dermatitis? Given the right circumstances, anyone can have combination skin. The designation is far too broad.

We have discussed oily and dry skin types. I make certain recommendations in the treatment of oily skin including the use of gentle cleansers and alcohol free toners. Regular exfoliation, hydration and UV protection are also helpful. People need to avoid excessively scrubbing their skin. If all the oil is stripped off, the skin gets a signal to make more.

With dry skin, avoidance of irritants and harsh soaps is important as is hydration and UV protection. The home should not be too dry and one should be cautious not to strip protective oils with products or long hot showers.

Remember, we are talking about skin "types" here. If someone has a certain facial distribution of acne, melasma or rosacea, that has nothing to do with skin 'type'. Those are skin *diseases*. Are some people more prone to get acne in the T-zone area? You bet, particularly those with oily skin.

In every chapter of this book I give my opinion based on research and my personal experience. I continue to learn and always check my thinking when my opinion seems to go against established standards of care. When I looked deeper, I found out that perhaps I was not alone in this combination skin question. If you search "combination skin" with The American Academy of Dermatology, Dermatology Times or Cutis.com there is not a single reference. Not one. Yet search the same on Google and 367,000 results show up. Every reference on the first page of results was selling a skin care product or a link to buying a skin care product. My primary concern with online discussions about combination skin is that there appears to be a strong push for the reader to first "think" they have combination skin then... buy something. If you dig deep, you can occasionally find discussion in regard to what could be *causing* changes in the texture, moisture level or oil content of the skin.

Another reason I question the term combination skin is because there is really nothing that unique about how it is treated with the exception of the common practice of keeping heavy moisturizers away from the T-zone area and perhaps being slightly more diligent about the exfoliation and cleansing of the T-zone. Even those recommendations aren't 'specific' to combination skin.

In fact, the common recommendations for combination skin include: the use of gentle cleansers, avoidance of harsh soaps, use of alcohol-free toners, UV ray protection, exfoliation, adequate hydration and the use of topical antioxidants. This is great advice for skin care, but is hardly specific to combination skin either. Avoidance of irritants is equally important for any skin type. Whether your skin is dry, normal, sensitive, or oily, if your approach to your skin results in irritation, I would suggest your skin type will change accordingly.

Essentially, my thought is that nobody's face is perfectly uniform in the distribution of sebaceous glands. If you have issues with your skin, *causes and conditions* need to be addressed first.

Despite the frequently discussed and debated topic of combination skin, It is my opinion that there are four skin types; normal, dry, oily and sensitive.

Age Spots

Age spots are also called "solar lentigines" or "liver spots". (As if they weren't bad enough without such a terrible name). These flat, tan, brown or black spots are caused by UV ray exposure and most commonly appear on the face, hands, shoulders, hands and arms. Age spots are very common in adults older than age 50 but may be present from the teen years on.

Age spots are quite unsightly and women tend to attempt to cover them up with makeup. Frequently this just makes matters worse.

The good news is age spots are benign (non-cancerous) and can be treated and prevented. Staying out of the sun or using sun block with SPF 20+ is a good start at preventing them from occurring in the first place. In some instances, however, you may want a doctor to look at them. This would be a case where a spot was very dark, was rapidly increasing in size, had an irregular border and/or a variable color pattern (i.e. variable color, pigment and border). I commonly suggest that *any* new spot you notice that is greater than 1 cm be checked by a doctor.

Where Do Age Spots Come From?

The pigment (melanin) in the upper layers of the skin (epidermis), gives the skin its normal color. People with dark complexions have more melanin and those of fair skin have less. In areas of the skin that have been subject to years of sun exposure, the melanin literally forms clumps which result in age spots. Other skin abnormalities such as a mole, keratosis, skin tag or psoriasis are raised above the skin surface. Age spots are not raised.

Treating Age Spots

The gold standard for treatment of age spots is intense pulsed light (IPL). The laser targets the melanin in the skin. This disrupts it and over the course of weeks it is sloughed to the surface. The best way to prevent age spots is through adequate use of sunblock. However, if the spots are already there, other options other than IPL are available.

LED treatments using green or red light have been proven beneficial in the fading of age spots. This is a strong alternative for someone hesitant to having an IPL.

Many topical treatments are also available which work to clear age spots. These will not clear them as quickly as having an IPL. However, they do help to clear age spots and help your skin in other ways as well.

- **Vitamin A (Retinol)** – As your skin's best friend, vitamin A unclogs pores, boosts collagen, and reduces inflammation. Its ability to speed up cell turnover helps to clear age spots.

- **Vitamin C** – This vitamin is well known for its antioxidant properties as well as its ability to reduce inflammation and clear unwanted pigment.

- **Hydroquinone** - through inhibition of the enzyme tyroinase hydroquinone effectively reduces visible pigment in the skin.

- **Niacinamide** - This fabulous vitamin improves the skin's barrier function, reduces inflammation and is an effective means of improving uneven skin texture and brown discolorations.

Once improvement is seen, a steady diet of sunblock, regular exfoliation and chemical peels will keep you skin looking its best.

Beautifying Your Eyes

Are your eyes giving your age away? Or even worse – making you look older than you actually are? Without a doubt, the area around your eyes is one of the very first areas of your face to succumb to aging. Studies have shown that upon meeting someone, people look first at a person's eyes ... then nose and mouth. Having dark circles, bags or wrinkles is not the first impression you want to give.

The subcutaneous fat (beneath the epidermis and dermis) serves as a type of cushion and support to these upper layers. The skin around the eye is very thin and delicate, containing very little of this subcutaneous fat. This fragile skin becomes even thinner as we age and hence more vulnerable to signs of aging. These changes commonly arrive as unwelcome dark circles, puffiness, fine lines and wrinkles. Let's take a look at some aging changes around the eyes and how we can reverse or prevent them, keeping your eyes youthful, clear and vibrant.

Dark Circles

Causes: Genetics / Poor Sleep / Allergies / Eye Irritation / UV rays

Genetics can play a role in literally any aging seen around the eyes. Dark circles are no exception. People with very fair skin tend to have even thinner-then-average skin around their eyes. When blood in tiny capillaries pools in this area under the eye it is much more noticeable in those with fair skin. When these capillaries are dilated it gives off a bluish hue. With poor sleep or stress, the problem is exacerbated. Fatigue causes the blood flow to become even more sluggish.

Seasonal allergies (and other allergies including food allergies) and chronic eye irritation cause the body to release a substance called *histamine*. Although the body is releasing histamine in an attempt to protect itself, around the eyes it simply causes further swelling of the blood vessels resulting in dark circles. People with chronic eye irritation from allergies or contact lenses make matters worse by *rubbing* that thin, delicate skin around the eye. UV rays contribute to the problem through an increase in the presence of free radicals and melanin secretion.

Dark Circle Treatments

1. Wear sunglasses – It's a great way to block those UV rays.
2. Sunblock – In terms of sunblock around the eye, it should contain zinc oxide or titanium oxide which will fully block the UV rays. These ingredients are also less likely to cause eye irritation.
3. Use a moisturizer with a *humectant* (like hyaluronic acid or glycerin) which will attract moisture to the area, plumping it up slightly so the capillaries are less visible.
4. Take an anti-histamine medication. Speak with your doctor first, but note that Claritin is over the counter and is probably one of the 'cleanest' medications out there in terms of giving tangible results with rare side effects. I have recommended it for years.
5. Use creams with brightening/pigment reducing agents. My favorites include niacinamide (vitamin B3), vitamin C, vitamin C-Ester, Hydroquinone and DMAE. These have been shown to fade excess melanin in the tissues as well as tighten the skin around the eye.
6. Have a medical aesthetic treatment. Dermal fillers to the tear trough area (under the eye) with fillers like Belotero or Restylane Silk can be very helpful as can LED light treatments. In terms of cosmetic lasers, the use of a Q-Switched 1,064nm

laser has been shown to be effective in the treatment of these dark circles.

Puffy and Baggy Eyes

Causes: Genetics, Diet (salt), Allergies, Alcohol, UV Rays

Some individuals have puffy eyes based on their genetics. They have larger fat pads around the eyes which can become more visible as they age. The skin around the eye is thin and delicate and will quickly reflect if one is retaining water (i.e. puffiness). Alcohol consumption and salty food are two other culprits causing fluid retention and puffy eyes. Stress and/or lack of sleep contribute as well.

Allergies and eye irritation can also exacerbate eye puffiness due to histamine release. UV rays cause more free radicals which can make eyes puffy and irritated. In some cases hormonal changes seen with menopause or hypothyroidism may be the cause.

In some fortunate people, gravity itself will help the puffiness resolve once their head is elevated in the morning. This is not always the case.

Puffy or Baggy Eye Treatments/Preventions

1. Diet - Avoiding alcohol and salty food is a start. Dietary choices can help even more. Foods that are high in anti-oxidants/anti-inflammatory ingredients like green leafy vegetables and vitamin A and C-rich fruits can be very beneficial. Seafood high in omega 3 fatty acids such as salmon and tuna are helpful as well.
2. Allergies or contact lens irritation: As noted above, in some people these allergies/irritations can cause dark circles. In others, the release of histamine results in swelling around the eye. Over the counter histamines can be very helpful in this regard, as can anti-histamine eye drops. Make sure you are following the optometrist's recommendation regarding cleaning and storing your contact lenses.

3. Sleep with your head elevated: Gravity is not the friend of those with puffy eyes. Some find sleeping on their back on two pillows to be helpful. Provided you can sleep comfortably in this position, it may be worth a try.

4. Hypothyroidism or hormonal changes: There indeed are more serious medical conditions with 'puffy eyes' showing up as a first symptom. It warrants investigation if your eyes have become puffy and remain so despite dietary changes. See your doctor. A simple blood test can determine if there are hormonal issues contributing to those puffy eyes.

5. Wash your makeup off before bed. Makeup around your eyes can cause eye irritation resulting in excessive puffiness in the morning.

6. Eye creams and serums: The use of creams and serums twice a day may be very helpful indeed. Choose one with ingredients such as aloe, vitamin E, retinol or DMAE.

7. Cool your eyes down: We are all familiar with spa pictures of a person with cucumber slices on their eyes. Whether it's a cucumber, tea bag or cold spoon, it is the cold that is helping the puffiness, not anything else. I am not a fan of tea bags or cucumbers due to potential infection. If you want to cool your eyes down, I prefer reusable gel eye masks that can be chilled and disinfected between uses.

8. Wear sunglasses and/or sunblock around the eye. Sunblock should contain zinc oxide or titanium oxide which will fully block the UV rays.

9. Surgical Options: If 1-8 above are not effective (which commonly is the case in those who have genetically large fat pads) speak to a cosmetic surgeon about blepharoplasty. This is a way to surgically correct droopy eyelids or bags under the eyes.

Fine Lines and Wrinkles

Causes: UV Rays, Genetics, Eye Strain

Every time you smile, laugh, squint, frown or yawn the small muscles around your eyes contract. In doing so, they are repeatedly scrunching the skin and collagen between them. Over the years, fine lines form and later become deep wrinkles. These creases fan out from the corner of your eye in the familiar 'crow's feet' distribution. Normal movement of the muscles around our eyes can be exacerbated by eye strain or squinting. UV rays and free radicals punish every layer of the skin making fine lines deeper.

Fine Line and Wrinkle Treatment:

1. Block UV rays in the form of sunglasses or sunblock containing zinc oxide or titanium oxide. I prefer SPF of 30+. Many people are very judicious about putting sunblock on their face and neck but miss the area around their eyes. Don't skip it.

2. Antioxidants – The use of alpha and beta hydroxy acids help remove dead skin cells and stimulate the growth of the supporting structures of collagen and elastin. Vitamin A (retinol) creams work similarly while speeding up cell turnover bringing fresher cells more quickly to the surface. Don't forget antioxidants in the diet in the form of green leafy vegetables, vitamin A and C-rich fruits and omega 3 fatty acid- rich seafood.

3. Medical Aesthetic Treatments: Botox Cosmetic has been the gold standard for treatment of crow's feet for 15 years. Through reversibly blocking nerve impulses the muscles around the eye do not contract and the area smoothens. Dysport and Xeomin work similarly. Other options include the injection of dermal fillers. For fine areas such as these, the use of Belotero and Restylane Silk has been successful. Other treatments such as microdermabrasion, chemical peels and microneedling can also improve the appearance of fine lines and wrinkles around the eye. Talk to your doctor or

aesthetician about which medical aesthetic treatment may be best for you.

Chapter Ten

Beauty and the Future

A Beauty Care Plan

A 37 year old woman came to me in a panic. She had made a last minute decision to attend her 20th class reunion. She looked in the mirror and wanted to look younger quickly. Time was of the essence. Similar situations may arise with an upcoming wedding or perhaps getting ready for a long week of holiday parties. Having a plan is important when you want to look your best with limited time.

I am not a proponent of the quick fix. However, I understand that there are times when treatments need to be approached aggressively and systematically to bring a quick, beautiful and natural result. Having a beauty care plan will help you understand how and when to have certain procedures done, what downtime to expect and a clear plan of action.

Beauty Phase 1 Treatments
Effective Anti-Aging Treatments Requiring Downtime

By no means do I suggest doing everything listed here. A solid plan would be to pick one or more procedure from each list and plan.

Microneedling:

Microneedling can be used on any skin type and it is less expensive than cosmetic laser treatments. Although the initial downtime (depending on the depth of the treatment) will be 3-7 days, the positive effects of microneedling will continue for a month or more as fibroblasts in the dermis continue to produce collagen and elastin to further tighten the skin. This is an effective anti-aging procedure to enhance your immediate beauty. If platelet rich plasma (PRP) is incorporated into your microneedling procedure more pronounced anti-aging effects may be achieved. Through the next 3-4 weeks there will be continued and steady improvement from this procedure.

About 7 days after this procedure you can move to Phase 2 treatments.

Laser Skin Resurfacing (Fraxel/Pixel):

Fraxel laser treatments make thousands of tiny holes through the epidermis into the dermis. There are areas of the skin between these holes that remain untouched. With holes going into the dermis, fibroblasts are stimulated to produce more collagen and elastin. This type of laser skin treatment helps to improve fine lines and wrinkles, acne scars or other scars while reducing the presence of age spots, freckles or other unwanted pigment. Your down time here is going to be perhaps as least as long, possibly longer as what is seen with microneedling. Typically one would need to wait 7-10 days after Fraxel before moving to Phase 2.

Intense Pulsed Light:

Intense Pulsed Light uses light energy to target chromophores in the skin. The light energy is converted to heat energy which damages and disrupts the architecture of the targeted cell. IPL is excellent for treatment of brown pigmented lesions (age spots), red discolorations (broken capillaries) as well as photo-rejuvenation of the skin through stimulation of fibroblasts to produce more collagen and elastin. IPL of course also can be used to remove unwanted hair. IPL can be combined in some cases with a Fraxel treatment. After IPL most can move to Phase 2 within a week.

Chemical Peels:

Chemical peels are divided into three broad categories; Superficial (light), medium and deep. In addition to beautiful exfoliation, deeper peels are able to clear unwanted pigment, improve acne (and acne scarring) and remove fine lines and wrinkles. Through penetration into the skin; through the epidermis and into the dermis, chemical peels help exfoliate, produce new and vibrant skin cells while stimulating dermal fibroblasts to make collagen and elastin. I would recommend a superficial or medium peel. A superficial peel really only requires a day or two of downtime (if that). With a medium peel, you may need to wait 5-7 days before moving to Phase 2.

Microdermabrasion

Microdermabrasion has a huge advantage over chemical peels and laser skin resurfacing in terms of down time and potential side effects. The main reason is because while giving a beautiful exfoliation, it doesn't penetrate beneath the epidermis.

Whether your aesthetician is using an aluminum oxide or diamond tip microdermabrasion system, the procedure will help to reduce fine lines and wrinkles, age spots, uneven pigment, minor scars or uneven skin texture. There is essentially no down time here and this can be done the day of, or one day before Phase 2 procedures.

A suggestion might be having an IPL, Fraxel or microneedling procedure. IPL could be *combined with* Fraxel or microneedling. A few weeks later have a microdermabrasion or light chemical peel. Less than a week after that, beauty Phase 2 treatments can begin.

Beauty Phase 2 Treatments
Dermal Fillers and Neurotoxins

Dermal Fillers

This is the first in your Phase 2 treatment plan. Dermal fillers, in the right hands really do not require any significant down time. Certainly there can be some redness and bruising, however it should be minimal if present at all. *Arnica,* in different forms, can be used to reduce the presence of bruising. Many times a 'touch up' may be needed which typically can be done 5-7 days after the initial treatment.

Neurotoxins

If you are in a pinch and want to see results quickly, the consensus is that Dysport has a faster onset of action (1-3 days) than Botox or Xeomin (both 3-5 days). Provided that the injector is not injecting Botox in the same location as the dermal filler, I typically have no issue with giving a neurotoxin like Botox the same day as injecting dermal fillers.

Skin Care Ingredients and Diet

Through Phases 1 and 2, it is of utmost importance to incorporate the right skin care ingredients along with your plan for beauty. The list of effective ingredients is long and needs to be tailored to what exactly you are trying to accomplish.

In terms of effective anti-aging ingredients, look for powerful antioxidants containing vitamin A, vitamin C, vitamin E, Green Tea, Resveratrol, Lycopene and Kojic Acid. The same holds true for diet. Antioxidant rich foods fight free radicals and keep your skin looking young and vibrant. Drinking plenty of water keeps the skin well hydrated.

Case Study: The 37 year old woman I mentioned had her reunion in 6 weeks. The only treatment she had ever come to me for was Botox. She clearly desired a more extensive plan this time.

She had many fine lines and wrinkles as well as age spots on her face and hands. There were dark circles under her eyes.

I started her on a skin care regimen of concentrated vitamin C-ester cream with DMAE to her face and neck along with hyaluronic acid face cream and alpha-lipoic-acid/vitamin C-ester eye cream. Her diet was to be items only from the Clear Skin diet; salmon, green leafy vegetables and vitamin A and C rich fruits and lots of water. We started with a full face and hand IPL followed by a full face Fraxel treatment. During the next 7-10 days she used a hyaluronic acid moisturizer followed by Agran oil (rich in essential fatty acids, vitamin and E). Then she returned to the previous skin care regimen.

Two weeks after her IPL/Fraxel she came in for a microdermabrasion and a light glycolic chemical peel. Week three she was in for Botox to her brow, forehead and crow's feet with a little in her chin to raise the corners of her mouth. I gave her Juvederm Ultra to her naso-labial folds, marionette lines and a touch of Restylane Silk in her tear troughs. I put 1.0 ml of Juvederm Voluma in each cheek. Week four was a touch up and week five was a quick microdermabrasion. Her 4-5 week transformation was complete. Her skin was clear and vibrant. She stated "I look 10 years younger than I did a month ago."

Having a solid plan for skin care and aesthetic treatments clearly works beautifully. The point here is not to recommend rushing in for many treatments. Rather, this case study should demonstrate that when you are coming in for medical aesthetic treatments, both you and your skin care professional should be thinking about moving toward your goals and taking deliberate, appropriate and effective steps to achieve them.

Medical Aesthetic Predictions

Change is inevitable. The day will come in the not-to-distant future when Botox will become obsolete. Seems impossible does it not? It will happen and while it may not be in the next 1-2 years …it is coming. This and other predictions I made were featured in LinkedIn Pulse and The Journal of Aesthetic Nursing.

#1 - Microneedling Challenges Laser Skin Resurfacing

Microneedling is not a new procedure by any means. The early dermal rollers of the 1990s have been replaced by newer electrical and battery powered devices. They actually do a much better job as well. Beverly Hills plastic surgeon Dr. Sheila Nazarian agrees stating the roller devices are, "sending needles in and out of your skin at an angle, actually nicking the skin as they come out, so it's causing more damage that you want."

The controlled skin injury here is something which bears similarity to Fraxel, but at a fraction of the cost. It is much easier for an office fit a microneedling device into their budget vs. a cosmetic laser which can cost tens of thousands of dollars.

Microneedling can treat many skin conditions and has become a hot topic on sites such as Real Self. The list of benefits of microneedling keeps growing. You will see a big increase in this procedure in the years ahead. Here is why:

1. It is an effective means to treat fine lines, wrinkles, loose skin, acne or other scarring, stretch marks, melasma or hyperpigmentation.
2. It is less expensive than laser skin resurfacing procedures like Fraxel and arguably equally or more effective. In an office questionnaire I found that people opted for microneedling over laser procedures because it offered "excellent results for less money."
3. There is far less downtime with microneedling vs. laser skin resurfacing.

4. Unlike chemical peels, microneedling can be used on any skin type.

A company called Endymed makes a product called the "Intensif RF" which beautifully combines microneedling and radiofrequency to give maximal results. It can be used to treat cellulite and stretch marks. Expect to see more of these treatments in the future, with newer devices incorporating more than one technology for skin rejuvenation.

The International Journal of Trichology showed 2 years ago that the use of, "Dermaroller along with Minoxidil was statistically superior to Minoxidil [alone] in promoting hair growth." More studies are being conducted and more patients are being treated for hair loss using microneedling technology. Essentially the list of benefits for microneedling keeps growing.

Microneedling is typically combined with the use of a wide array of skin care ingredients to increase the effectiveness and absorption of these products. For instance: Vitamin C (collagen), hydroquinone (pigment), vitamin A (skin rejuvenation and acne), peptides (collagen) and platelet rich plasma.

This brings us to prediction #2.

#2 – Neuropeptides Challenge Botox

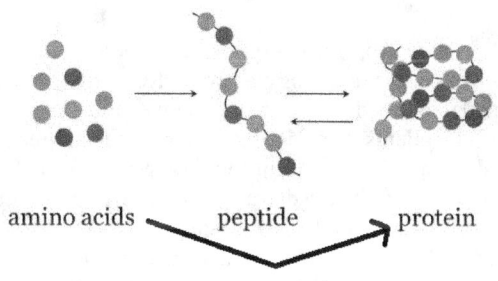

amino acids   peptide   protein

In the discussion of peptides we discussed signal peptides, copper peptides and neuropeptides.

When protein is broken down, peptides are formed. These peptides can combine with amino acids to form more protein. The fact that peptides are present, however, serves as a signal that collagen has been broken down and needs to be replaced. Therefore, more peptides mean a stronger signal for your body (skin) to make more protein (collagen). Applying peptides directly to your skin thereby tricks your skin into making more collagen. The most popular 'signal' peptide seen in skin care is Palmitoyl Pentapeptide.

Neuropeptides vs. Botox

Neuropeptides are peptides that play a role in nerve cell communication. Botox binds to facial nerves to ultimately prevent contraction of facial muscles. A neuropeptide known as argireline may block the release of neurotransmitters from nerves. In theory, if absorbed all the way to the level of the muscle, it may block contraction of the muscle leading to smoother skin, much like Botox. Expect to see more research and studies aiming to prove neuropeptides can do what Botox does. If it does not happen in this year or two, mark my words, the day that a skin cream or serum can be applied to the face to give results similar to Botox, is coming quickly. Botox, by a huge margin is #1. It will be challenged. Nobody stays on top forever.

#3 – Medical Aesthetics – Apps and Telemedicine Arrive

There seems to be an App for everything and the medical spa arena will see growth in this technology as well. Recently, Modiface and Allergan Canada released a live facial rejuvenation app. Here the technology offers clients considering different facial treatments to view projected results. Do you want to know what you will look like following a treatment with Juvederm? This app will allow this along with views from multiple angles. This is a game changer and will do nothing but increase the already staggering growth of the medical aesthetics industry. I foresee that offices will either incorporate apps like this or newer ones along with a real-time telemedicine encounter.

Here is what is coming: You go to a medical spa website or go through the medical spa app. You use the app you see how your face will look before and after specific treatments (for instance – 1ml of Restylane to each nasolabial fold). Then, you will be able to have a telemedicine ('real time') face to face online consult with a skin care professional to discuss options, treatments, cost, and to book an appointment. The medical spa and surgery centers at the forefront of this technology will stand out as leaders in the industry.

Before discussing number 4 and 5, it is worth noting that in terms of cosmetic surgery (*surgical* procedures performed), the 2015 data from the American Society of Plastic Surgeons showed:

Cosmetic Surgical Procedures 2015		
Procedure	Number Performed	Change since 2014
Breast Augmentation	286,254	Down 1%
Nose Reshaping	217,124	Down 2%
Liposuction	210,552	**UP 5%**
Eyelid Surgery	206,509	Down 4%
Facelift	128,266	Down 4%

Liposuction and facelifts remain huge markets for cosmetic surgeons and made up 33% of surgical procedures in 2015. This is important because these two areas will continue to show tremendous growth in the **non-surgical** arena.

#4 – Increase in Non-Surgical Fat Reduction Procedures

When it comes to non-surgical fat reduction, big players in this market include Coolsculpting, Quantashape, Liposonix, Vanquish RF and Alma Accent.

According to a survey performed by the American Society for Dermatologic Surgery, up to **65%** of people said they have a level of dissatisfaction with under-the-chin fullness. Coolsculpting, for example, essentially freezes stubborn fat cells, which the body then disposes of through the lymphatic system. The treatment is performed by placing an applicator on the treatment area, which attaches via vacuum suction, and gradually freezes the targeted fat over a 60-minute session. Patients may need to undergo a course of treatments to achieve their desired results, but many report seeing results after a single session.

Fat and Cellulite Treatments 2016	
Coolsculpting	Controlled Cooling (cryolipolysis)
Quantashape	Ultrasound plus "zonal massage"
Liposonix	High Intensity Focused Ultrasound (HIFU)
Ultrashape	High Intensity Focused Ultrasound (HIFU)
Vanquish RF	Radiofrequency
Accent XL	Radiofrequency
Velashape	Radiofrequency / Infrared / Massage
Kybella	Cryolipolysis (injection)

Says Dr. Vitenas, plastic surgeon from Houston, "Seven different CoolSculpting attachments are available; each made to treat a different area of the body. The most commonly addressed areas with CoolSculpting include the abdomen, lower back, upper arms, chin and the thighs."

In September of 2015 the FDA approved the Coolsculpting "CoolMini" for treatment of the area under the chin. The CoolMini while designed for submental fat (under the chin) can also be used on hard to treat areas. The CoolMini successfully eliminates layers of fatty tissue below the chin, leaving the jawline smooth and taut.

Kybella is not a laser. It is a product that is injected, dissolving the fat cell's membrane to effectively kill the cell, which is then cleared through the body's lymphatic system. This procedure is much quicker than a coolsculpting treatment. However, with Kybella it is important to note that results are *highly injector dependent*. Says Stephanie Hill (expert Kybella injector and trainer), "Kybella gives consistent results to anyone searching for a permanent reduction of (submental) chin fat." Expect to see more medical aesthetic doctors training to perform this procedure in the future as well. The future is bright for Kybella indeed.

#5 – More Non-Surgical Face Lifts

Dermal filler use has nearly doubled in the past 5 years (a 94% increase). Expect this to continue along with an increased use of deeper dermal injections for cheek and mid-face augmentation.

Products such as Radiesse, Juvederm Voluma and Restylane Lyft will continue to have a strong showing in the near future due to the unique attributes of these products. Specifically they have a larger molecular size, more cross-linking and a higher G-prime. These bulkier, 'stickier' fillers have the ability (when injected properly) to give a true lift particularly to the areas of the cheeks and mid face.

The State of the Medical Aesthetic Industry

Women have always wanted to look and feel beautiful. However, as we enter the second half of this decade, the rules have changed. We have now entered into what I would refer to as 'The Era of Beauty.' This era is a product of the evolution of procedures offered in the realm of medical aesthetics.

The medical aesthetic industry continues to experience a feverish rate of growth. The broad acceptance and cost-effective nature of procedures are at the core of this prosperity.

A study by Allergan beautifully illustrated and clarified why this growth is occurring. Of women surveyed 83% revealed that they "wanted to look as natural as possible in order to better reflect their personalities, expressions and emotional well-being." This goal does not align with aggressive plastic surgery. To me, this means the subtle changes one can experience with a visit to a medical spa for a neurotoxin (Botox), dermal filler, chemical peel, microdermabrasion, microneedling or laser procedure. That is what people want. Subtle youthful and beautiful results are what they get. And they keep coming back for more.

Aestheticians Needed

There are currently about 40,000 Aestheticians in the United States. It comes as no surprise that this job market is expected to increase 39.8% between 2012 and 2022. The majority of positions for aestheticians are in California, Texas, New York, Arizona and Oregon. The average salary is $33,810 with the top 10% making $58,000 or more/year. High compensation was seen in the metropolitan areas of Albuquerque, New Mexico, Washington, D.C. and Portland, Oregon.

Medical Aesthetics MD, DO, DDS, etc.

Fifteen years ago the only doctors performing aesthetic procedures were cosmetic surgeons and dermatologists. Not so in 2016. Primary care doctors are experiencing increased frustration and burnout. The reduced autonomy, increased paperwork, battles with insurance companies and 70 hour work weeks have taken their toll on these well-intentioned doctors.

Said one Minnesota physician, "I can do a laser treatment for $1500 which is slightly less than what I charge for full pregnancy care (which I must fight with insurers to collect)."

Beware the You Tube Specialist

I was training a physician on the use of Botox and dermal fillers and explained to him bluntly, "You realize, since you have an 'MD' after your name technically you are licensed to inject Botox." He understood my point. This doctor was learning how to inject Botox the *right way*. Before he stuck a single needle into someone's face, he was making sure he knew every nuance in regard to Botox's mechanism of action, potential side effects and results to be achieved.

Every doctor is not necessarily like this one. With the ever expanding library of YouTube, many professionals are taking ill-advised short cuts in their quest to make a quick medical aesthetic buck. I will grant you that many of the videos are very descriptive and well done, but would you really want a doctor with a medical degree from an online medical school? Having hands on training and practice is vital to assuring safe and effective medical aesthetic results, no exceptions.

Any medical aesthetic procedure in the right hands can and will give amazing results. In the hands of an untrained or poorly trained professional, these simple procedures suddenly become downright dangerous.

A final caution is a big sale in a new medical spa. Sure it is understandable that a new spa would like to entice new clients. However, if the first thing that draws you to a medical spa is a sale, you are off to a terrible start. Listen, if you are buying a new pair of jeans and they are on sale that is one thing, a sale on someone hitting your face with a laser or putting a needle next to your eye is another.

My Take on it All

Medical Aesthetics is an amazing field and if you are considering entering as an aesthetician, nurse or physician, you are hitting it at a fantastic time.

For those considering an aesthetic procedure, beyond using common sense my recommendations are:

1. By and large, you get what you pay for.

2. Ask to see credentials and licenses. There should *never* be an issue or uncomfortable moment about this question.

3. Attend a conference. Getting connected in the industry is an excellent way to assure you know the best treatments available and just what questions to ask when you walk into that medical-spa.

4. Buy my next book or visit me at ClearSkinMD.net. I am a true patient advocate and that equates to education and empowerment of patients considering treatments of any kind.

In Closing

What has transpired over the past decade in the world of medical aesthetics is astounding. My desire to remain in the forefront of this field is multifactorial. Being in a position to help people look and feel better, while improving their self-esteem is a role I hold near and dear to my heart. I am fortunate to have been able to do so. Another reason is as technology improves, the way I am able to help people look and feel better improves as well.

Before 1928, there were no antibiotics. Doctors were very limited in what they could do to help people with infections. Pneumonia would kill many people. Now, it is frequently treated by a visit to the doctor or urgent care center and handled quite commonly on an outpatient basis. That is amazing. I see medical aesthetics in a similar way. True, it is not life or death but its importance cannot be underestimated. What seemed impossible 20 years ago is literally main-stream today.

People will always want to look and feel better if possible. When Botox came along, there was a huge shift in the thinking of the public and professionals. People could now take a more active role in making huge anti-aging strides. Hyaluronic acid dermal fillers were the next big leap. With new lasers treatments coming available and continued improvement to the existing products, the future is nothing less than amazing in this field.

Each step you take toward anti-aging through skin care, medical aesthetic treatments, diet or exercise brings you one step closer to a younger and more beautiful you.

Watch for *Volume II of Winning Skin* coming in the summer of 2017. In the meantime you are always welcome to visit me at ClearSkinMD.net

Be well and be good to your skin.

References

Chapter 1

1. Vanderbilt University psychologist, David Schlundt
    http://www.vanderbilt.edu/psychological_sciences/bio/david-schlundt
2. Vivian Diller, PhD
    http://www.viviandiller.com/
3. "Average American Woman's Height and Weight," Adam Cole, Livestrong.com, 10/27/2015.
4. Federal Reserve Bank of St. Louis
    https://www.stlouisfed.org/publications/regional-economist/october-2011/worth-your-weight-reexamining-the-link-between-obesity-and-wages
5. Heather Patrick – Research – National Institutes of Health
    http://blog.creativelive.com/what-beauty-means/

Chapter 2

1. Dean M. Tomasello, MD "Independent Survey-Initial Aesthetics", Dean Michael Aesthetics 11/2010.
2. James P. Bonaparte, MD, *JAMA Facial Plastic Surgery*, May 2015, http://media.jamanetwork.com/news-item/pliability-elasticity-of-skin-increase-following-wrinkle-treatment-with-botox/
3. "Relationship between Physical Activity Level, Telomere Length and Telomerase Activity" Medicine and Science in Sports and Exercise, October, 2008, http://www.ncbi.nlm.nih.gov/pmc/articles/PMC2581416/
4. "Prevalence of Health Sleep Duration among Adults," CDC, February, 2016
    http://www.cdc.gov/mmwr/volumes/65/wr/mm6506a1.htm

Chapter 3

1. NIH, "Free radicals, antioxidants and functional foods: Impact on human health"
   http://www.ncbi.nlm.nih.gov/pmc/articles/PMC3249911/
2. Journal of Dermatologic Surgery, July, 2005
   http://onlinelibrary.wiley.com/doi/10.1111/j.1524-4725.2005.31732/abstract
3. National Institutes of Health, Free radicals
   http://www.ncbi.nlm.nih.gov/pmc/articles/PMC3249911/
4. Clinical Interventions in Aging, 2006, Retinol
   http://www.ncbi.nlm.nih.gov/pmc/articles/PMC2699641/
5. Vitamin C-Ester, Perricone, MD, "The Wrinkle Cure," p. 61-66.
6. "Why don't we use Vitamin E in dermatology" CMAJ, November, 1993
   http://www.ncbi.nlm.nih.gov/pmc/articles/PMC1485678/
7. Dietary vs. Topical Green Tea
   http://www.smartskincare.com/treatments/topical/greentea.html
8. Resveratrol https://en.wikipedia.org/wiki/Resveratrol
9. Achives of Biochemistry and Biophysics 2011, Resveratrol
   http://www.ncbi.nlm.nih.gov/pmc/articles/PMC3060966/
10. Alpha Lipoic Acid, Perricone, MD, "The Wrinkle Cure," p.67-80.
11. Niacinamide improves skin barrier in patients with Rosacea
    http://www.ncbi.nlm.nih.gov/pubmed/16209160
12. Niacinamide improves dry skin, International Journal of Dermatology, March, 2005
    http://www.ncbi.nlm.nih.gov/pubmed/15807725
13. "Topical nicotinamide compared with clindamycin gel in the treatment of inflammatory acne vulgaris," International Journal of Dermatology, June, 1995
    http://www.ncbi.nlm.nih.gov/pubmed/7657446
14. "Argan Oil leads to the inhibition of tyrosinase" The Journal of Evidence Based Complementary and Alternative Medicine,

July 8, 2013
http://www.ncbi.nlm.nih.gov/pmc/articles/PMC3723062/
15. "Grape Seed Extract," Global Journal of Health Science 2014
http://search.proquest.com/openview/7ef5afc36f7b44402baa45
92d30128f6/1?pq-origsite=gscholarr
16. OPCs, Grape seed extract
http://www.ncbi.nlm.nih.gov/pubmed/14977436
17. FDA Organic labeling in cosmetics
http://www.fda.gov/Cosmetics/Labeling/Claims/ucm203078.ht
m

Chapter 4

1. "Review of Exfoliating Devices", Dean M. Tomasello, MD,
ClearSkinMD.net, 2/9/2016,
https://www.clearskinmd.net/exfoliating-devices/
2. 2014 Plastic Surgery Statistics Report
http://www.plasticsurgery.org/Documents/news-
resources/statistics/2014-statistics/plastic-surgery-statsitics-full-
report.pdf
3. Kybella and Kybella patient satisfaction, April, 2105
https://globenewswire.com/news-
release/2015/04/29/730181/10131585/en/Photo-Release-
KYTHERA-Biopharmaceuticals-Announces-FDA-Approval-of-
KYBELLA-TM-also-known-as-ATX-101-First-and-Only-
Submental-Contouring-Injectable-Drug.html
4. Chin Liposuction average cost https://www.realself.com/Chin-
liposuction/reviews
5. Coolsculpting, excerpts courtesy of Dr. Paul Vitenas
http://www.drvitenas.com/
6. Kybella, excerpts courtesy of Sean Johnson, MBA
7. Melasma treatment with Red Light LED, The American Journal
of Dermatology and Venereology, September, 2014
8. Psoriasis treatment with Red Light LED, Seminars in Cutaneous
Medicine and Surgery (Aug 2014)
9. Journal of Depression and Anxiety, 2009, Blue light and
seasonal affective disorder Depression and Anxiety volume 26,

Issue   3   pp.273-278.
http://onlinelibrary.wiley.com/doi/10.1002/da.20538/abstract

Chapter 5

1. Food and Nutrition Board, February 2004,
   http://www.nationalacademies.org/hmd/Reports/2004/Dietary-
   Reference-Intakes-Water-Potassium-Sodium-Chloride-and-
   Sulfate.aspx
2. "Water, Hydration and Health," Nutritional Review, August,
   2010, http://www.ncbi.nlm.nih.gov/pmc/articles/PMC2908954/
3. "What is a serving," American Heart Association, February,
   2015,
   http://www.heart.org/HEARTORG/Caregiver/Replenish/Whatis
   aServing/What-is-a-
   Serving_UCM_301838_Article.jsp#.VvA7IdIrKM8
4. "Food Allergies", excerpts taken from www.foodallergy.org
5. "Polypodium leucotomos as an Adjunct Treatment of
   Pigmentary Disorders, Journal of Clinical and Aesthetic
   Dermatology, March, 2014.
   http://www.ncbi.nlm.nih.gov/pubmed/24688621
6. "The effect of an oral supplement containing glucosamine
   amino acids, minerals and antioxidants on cutaneous aging: a
   preliminary study," Journal of Dermatological Treatment,
   Volume 12, Issue 1, 2001.
   http://www.tandfonline.com/doi/abs/10.1080/095466301750163
   590?journalCode=ijdt20
7. Ellen Murmur, MD, author and professor of Dermatology at Mt.
   Sinai School of Medicine.
   http://feelingfit.com/beauty/topic/9107-40/story

Chapter 6

1. Botulinum Toxin, Alastair and Jean Carruthers
   http://www.revance.com/pdfs/Waugh-Topical-Neurotoxin-
   Procedures-in-Cosmetic-Dermatology-3rd-Edition.pdf
2. "Pliability, Elasticity of Skin Increase Following Wrinkle
   Treatment with Botox," James P. Bonaparte, MD,

http://media.jamanetwork.com/news-item/pliability-elasticity-of-skin-increase-following-wrinkle-treatment-with-botox/

3. "Factors that motivate people to undergo cosmetic surgery," Canadian Journal of Plastic Surgery, Winter, 2012.
http://www.ncbi.nlm.nih.gov/pmc/articles/PMC3513261/

4. "Duration of Action of AbobotulinumtoxinA and OnabotulinumtoxinA," Journal of Clinical and Aesthetic Dermatology, September, 2011.
http://www.ncbi.nlm.nih.gov/pmc/articles/PMC3175804/

5. "What is off label use? A doctor explains," New Beauty, Shellie Terry Benson, Feburary 24, 2012.
https://www.newbeauty.com/hottopic/blogpost/1384-what-is-off-label-use-a-doctor-explains/

Chapter 7

1. "Filler lift a result of more than G-Prime," The Dermatology Times, April 1, 2014.
http://dermatologytimes.modernmedicine.com/dermatology-times/news/filler-lift-result-more-g-prime

2. "Soft Tissue Fillers Approved by the Center for Devices and Radiological Health," FDA.gov,
http://www.fda.gov/MedicalDevices/ProductsandMedicalProcedures/CosmeticDevices/WrinkleFillers/ucm227749.htm

3. Voluma Briefing Book by Allergan, Inc. April 4 2014,
http://www.fda.gov/ucm/groups/fdagov-public/@fdagov-afda-adcom/documents/document/ucm349428.pdf

4. "Guide to Sculptra," SkinTour,
http://www.skintour.com/fillers-botox-injectibles/dermal-fillers-juvederm-restylane-sculptra-radiesse/guide-to-sculptra/

5. "Hand recontouring with calcium hydroxylapatitie (Radiesse)," Journal of Cosmetic Dermatology, March 2009.
http://www.ncbi.nlm.nih.gov/pubmed/19250166

6. BLT Cream is effective prior to laser or cosmetic procedures, Cosmetic Dermatology April, 2003.

Chapter 8

1. 2014 medical aesthetic statistics
   http://www.plasticsurgery.org/Documents/news-resources/statistics/2014-statistics/plastic-surgery-statsitics-full-report.pdf
2. "Money women and men spend for cosmetic procedures"
   http://www.dailymail.co.uk/femail/article-2417796/The-average-woman-spend-18-000-face-lifetime.html
3. Success of Vaniqua Treatments
   http://www.accessdata.fda.gov/drugsatfda_docs/label/2000/21145lbl.pdf
4. Coolsculpting – Excerpts courtesy of Dr. Paul Vitenas
5. "Current trends in Intense Pulsed Light," The Journal of Clinical and Aesthetic Dermatology, June 2012.
   http://www.ncbi.nlm.nih.gov/pmc/articles/PMC3390232/
6. "Fractionated bipolar radiofrequency devices rejuvenate the skin," Dermatology Times, 2/9/15.
   http://dermatologytimes.modernmedicine.com/dermatology-times/news/fractionated-bipolar-radiofrequency-devices-rejuvenate-skin?page=full
7. Laser Tattoo Removal, "The Consulting Room"
   http://www.consultingroom.com/treatment/laser-tattoo-removal
8. Statistic Brain   http://www.statisticbrain.com/tattoo-statistics

Chapter 9

1. Journal of Clinical and Aesthetic dermatology
   http://www.ncbi.nlm.nih.gov/pmc/articles/PMC3013592/
2. Medical Journal of Australia – Tea Tree oil
   http://www.ncbi.nlm.nih.gov/pmc/articles/PMC1360273/
3. Oily Skin – American Journal of Clinical Dermatology, 2009, vol. 10
4. Oily Skin – Journal of Investigative Dermatology, November 2006.

5. WebMD / Combination Skin.
   http://www.webmd.com/beauty/face/whats-your-skin-type

Chapter 10

1. Beverly Hills plastic surgeon Dr. Sheila Nazarian
   http://nazarianplasticsurgery.com/dermapen-micro-needling/
2. International Journal of Trichology
   http://www.ncbi.nlm.nih.gov/pmc/articles/PMC3746236/
3. Modiface/Allergan Canada
   http://modiface.com/news.php?story=610
4. American Society for Dermatologic Surgery
   https://www.asds.net/
5. "Coolsculpting" courtesy Dr. Paul Vitenas. www.drvitenas.com
6. FDA Coolscupting approval.
   http://investor.coolsculpting.com/releasedetail.cfm?releaseid=932755
7. Women and Natural Beauty, PRNewswire,
   http://www.prnewswire.co.uk/news-releases/changing-face-of-beauty-women-want-to-look-natural-153575815.html
8. Kybella, Non-Surgical Fat Reduction,
   Courtesy Stephanie Hill, Clinical Assistant
   http://www.worldofaesthetics.com
9. Aesthetician Job Market, Sokanu,
   https://www.sokanu.com/careers/aesthetician/jobs/